PAIN MEDICINE
A CASE-BASED LEARNING SERIES

The Shoulder and Elbow

The Spine
9780323756365

 The Hip and Pelvis
9780323762977

 The Knee
9780323762588

 Headache and Facial Pain
9780323834568

 The Wrist and Hand
9780323834537

 The Chest Wall and Abdomen
9780323846882

 The Ankle and Foot
9780323870382

PAIN MEDICINE
A CASE-BASED LEARNING SERIES

The Shoulder and Elbow

STEVEN D. WALDMAN, MD, JD

ELSEVIER

Elsevier
1600 John F. Kennedy Blvd.
Ste 1800
Philadelphia, PA 19103-2899

PAIN MEDICINE: A CASE-BASED LEARNING SERIES ISBN: 978-0-323-75877-2
THE SHOULDER AND ELBOW

Notice

Library of Congress Control Number: 2021936720

Executive Content Strategist: Michael Houston
Content Development Specialist: Jeannine Carrado/Laura Klien
Director, Content Development: Ellen Wurm-Cutter
Publishing Services Manager: Shereen Jameel
Senior Project Manager: Karthikeyan Murthy
Design Direction: Amy Buxton

Printed in India

Last digit is the print number: 9 8 7 6 5 4 3 2

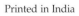
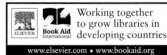

Working together
to grow libraries in
developing countries

www.elsevier.com • www.bookaid.org

To Peanut and David H.

SDW

"When you go after honey with a balloon, the great thing is to not let the bees know you're coming."

WINNIE THE POOH

It's Harder Than It Looks
MAKING THE CASE FOR CASE-BASED LEARNING

For sake of full disclosure, I was one of those guys. You know, the ones who wax poetic about how hard it is to teach our students how to do procedures. Let me tell you, teaching folks how to do epidurals on women in labor certainly takes its toll on the coronary arteries. It's true, I am amazing...I am great...I have nerves of steel. Yes, I could go on like this for hours...but you have heard it all before. But, it's again that time of year when our new students sit eagerly before us, full of hope and dreams...and that harsh reality comes slamming home...it is a lot harder to teach beginning medical students "doctoring" than it looks.

A few years ago, I was asked to teach first-year medical and physician assistant students how to take a history and perform a basic physical exam. In my mind I thought "this should be easy...no big deal". I won't have to do much more than show up. After all, I was the guy who wrote that amazing book on physical diagnosis. After all, I had been teaching medical students, residents, and fellows how to do highly technical (and dangerous, I might add) interventional pain management procedures since right after the Civil War. Seriously, it was no big deal...I could do it in my sleep...with one arm tied behind my back...blah...blah...blah.

For those of you who have had the privilege of teaching "doctoring," you already know what I am going to say next. *It's harder than it looks!* Let me repeat this to disabuse any of you who, like me, didn't get it the first time. *It is harder than it looks!* I only had to meet with my first-year medical and physician assistant students a couple of times to get it through my thick skull: **It really is harder than it looks**. In case you are wondering, the reason that our students look back at us with those blank, confused, bored, and ultimately dismissive looks is simple: They lack context. That's right, they lack the context to understand what we are talking about.

It's really that simple...or hard...depending on your point of view or stubbornness, as the case may be. To understand why context is king, you have to look only as far as something as basic as the Review of Systems. The Review of Systems is about as basic as it gets, yet why is it so perplexing to our students? Context. I guess it should come as no surprise to anyone that the student is completely lost when you talk about...let's say...the "constitutional" portion of the Review of Systems, without the context of what a specific constitutional finding, say a fever or chills, might mean to a patient who is suffering from the acute onset of headaches. If you tell the student that you need to ask about fever, chills, and the other "constitutional" stuff and you take it no further, you might as well be talking about the

International Space Station. Just save your breath; it makes absolutely no sense to your students. Yes, they want to please, so they will memorize the elements of the Review of Systems, but that is about as far as it goes. On the other hand, if you present the case of Jannette Patton, a 28-year-old first-year medical resident with a fever and headache, you can see the lights start to come on. By the way, this is what Jannette looks like, and as you can see, Jannette is sicker than a dog. This, at its most basic level, is what *Case-Based Learning* is all about.

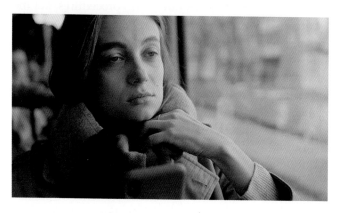

I would like to tell you that, smart guy that I am, I immediately saw the light and became a convert to *Case-Based Learning*. But truth be told, it was COVID-19 that really got me thinking about *Case-Based Learning*. Before the COVID-19 pandemic, I could just drag the students down to the med/surg wards and walk into a patient room and riff. Everyone was a winner. For the most part, the patients loved to play along and thought it was cool. The patient and the bedside was all I needed to provide the context that was necessary to illustrate what I was trying to teach—the why headache and fever don't mix kind of stuff. Had COVID-19 not rudely disrupted my ability to teach at the bedside, I suspect that you would not be reading this *Preface*, as I would not have had to write it. Within a very few days after the COVID-19 pandemic hit, my days of bedside teaching disappeared, but my students still needed context. This got me focused on how to provide the context they needed. The answer was, of course, *Case-Based Learning*. What started as a desire to provide context. . .because it really was **harder than it looked**. . .led me to begin work on this eight-volume *Case-Based Learning* textbook series. What you will find within these volumes are a bunch of fun, real-life cases that help make each patient come alive for the student. These cases provide the contextual teaching points that make it easy for the teacher to explain why, when Jannette's chief complaint is, *"My head is killing me and I've got a fever,"* it is a big deal.

Have fun!

Steven D. Waldman, MD, JD
Spring 2021

ACKNOWLEDGMENTS

A very special thanks to my editors, Michael Houston, PhD, Jeannine Carrado, and Karthikeyan Murthy, for all of their hard work and perseverance in the face of disaster. Great editors such as Michael, Jeannine, and Karthikeyan make their authors look great, for they not only understand how to bring the Three Cs of great writing...Clarity + Consistency + Conciseness...to the author's work, but unlike me, they can actually punctuate and spell!

Steven D. Waldman, MD, JD

P.S. ...Sorry for all the ellipses, guys!

CONTENTS

Bill Kidder

A 58-Year-Old Male With Right Shoulder Pain

LEARNING OBJECTIVES

- Learn the common causes of shoulder pain.
- Develop an understanding of the unique anatomy of the shoulder joint.
- Develop an understanding of the causes of glenohumeral joint arthritis.
- Learn the clinical presentation of osteoarthritis of the glenohumeral joint.
- Learn how to use physical examination to identify pathology of the rotator cuff.
- Develop an understanding of the treatment options for osteoarthritis of the glenohumeral joint.
- Learn the appropriate testing options to help diagnose osteoarthritis of the glenohumeral joint.
- Learn to identify red flags waving in patients who present with shoulder pain.
- Develop an understanding of the role in interventional pain management in the treatment of shoulder pain.

Bill Kidder

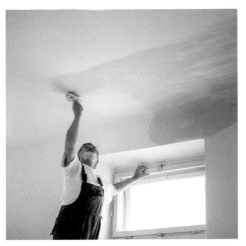

Bill Kidder is a 58-year-old painter with the chief complaint of "my right shoulder is killing me." Bill went on to say that he wouldn't have bothered coming in, but he was getting where he couldn't paint ceilings anymore. I asked Bill if he had anything like this happen before. He shook his head and responded, "Just the usual aches that a guy my age comes to expect. You can't work all day as a painter and not have some pain. Usually I just take a couple of Motrin and use a heating pad. That will usually set me right after a day or so. What worries me this time is that this damn right shoulder is hurting all the time, especially when I reach up to cut in the top of a wall or paint a ceiling. I'm pretty tough, but this has me worried because if I don't work, I don't eat. The other thing is, this damn shoulder has my sleep all jacked up. Every time I roll over on it, the damn pain wakes me up! Hell, some mornings I can't even comb my hair."

I asked Bill about any antecedent trauma and he just shook his head. "Doc, this kind of snuck up on me. At first, my shoulder had this deep ache that would get better with some Motrin and rest. Over time, the Motrin just quit working. But Doc, like I said, I gotta work." I asked Bill what made his pain worse and he said, "Any time I use this shoulder, it hurts."

I asked Bill to point with one finger to show me where it hurts the most. He grabbed his right shoulder and said, "Doc, I can't really point to one place, it kind of hurts all over; and you know Doc, the crazy thing is, sometimes I feel like the shoulder is popping." I asked if he had any fever or chills and he shook his head no. "What about steroids? Did you ever take any cortisone or drugs like that, Bill?" Bill again shook his head no, then said, "Doc, you know me. I am healthy as a horse. If it wasn't for this damn shoulder, I'd arm-wrestle you!" I laughed and said I'd take a raincheck on the arm wrestle, but after I got his shoulder better "we would see who was the better man!" Bill smiled and said, "Doc, you're on!"

On physical examination, Bill was afebrile. His respirations were 18 and his pulse was 74 and regular. His blood pressure (BP) was slightly elevated at 142/84. I made a note to recheck it again before he left because who knew when or if he would come back. His head, eyes, ears, nose, throat (HEENT) exam was normal, as was his cardiopulmonary examination. His thyroid was normal. His abdominal examination revealed no abnormal mass or organomegaly. There

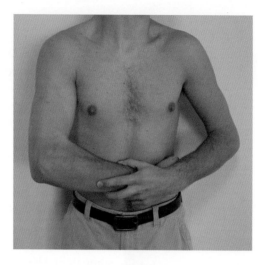

Fig. 1.1   Visual inspection of the shoulder. (From Waldman SD. *Physical Diagnosis of Pain: An Atlas of Signs and Symptoms*. 3rd ed. St Louis, MO: Elsevier; 2016 [Fig. 18.1].)

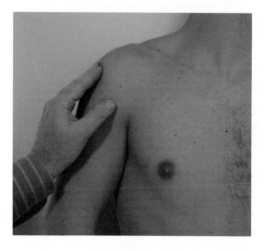

Fig. 1.2   Palpation of the shoulder. (From Waldman SD. *Physical Diagnosis of Pain: An Atlas of Signs and Symptoms*. 3rd ed. St Louis, MO: Elsevier; 2016 [Fig. 19.1].)

was no costovertebral angle (CVA) tenderness. There was no peripheral edema. His low back examination was unremarkable. I did a rectal exam, which revealed no mass and a normal prostate. Visual inspection of the right shoulder revealed no cutaneous lesions or obvious mass (Fig. 1.1). The shoulder was cool to touch. Palpation of the right shoulder revealed mild diffuse tenderness, with no obvious effusion or point tenderness (Fig. 1.2). There was mild crepitus, but I did not

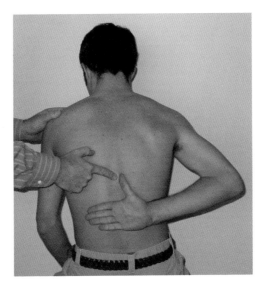

Fig. 1.3 Internal rotation of the shoulder. (From Waldman S. *Physical Diagnosis of Pain: An Atlas of Signs and Symptoms*. 3rd ed. St Louis, MO: Elsevier; 2016 [Fig. 21.1].)

appreciate any popping. Range of motion was decreased, with pain exacerbated with elevation and internal rotation of the shoulder (Fig. 1.3). The drop test was negative bilaterally (Fig. 1.4). The left shoulder examination was normal, as was examination of his other major joints, other than some mild osteoarthritis in the right hand. A careful neurologic examination of the upper extremities revealed that there was no evidence of peripheral or entrapment neuropathy, and the deep tendon reflexes were normal.

Key Clinical Points—What's Important and What's Not

THE HISTORY

- No history of acute trauma
- No history of previous significant shoulder pain
- No fever or chills
- Gradual onset of shoulder pain, with exacerbation of pain with shoulder use
- Popping sensation in the right shoulder
- Sleep disturbance
- Difficulty elevating the affected upper extremity to comb hair or paint ceilings

THE PHYSICAL EXAMINATION

- The patient is afebrile
- Normal visual inspection of shoulder

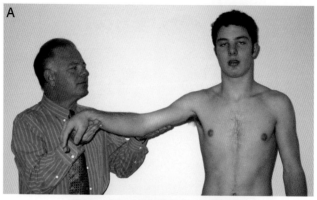

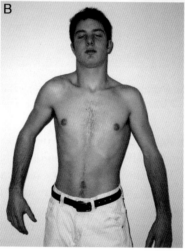

Fig. 1.4 (A, B) The drop arm test for complete rotator cuff tear. (From Waldman S. *Physical Diagnosis of Pain: An Atlas of Signs and Symptoms*. 3rd ed. St Louis, MO: Elsevier; 2016 [Figs. 52.1 and 52.2].)

- Palpation of right shoulder reveals diffuse tenderness
- No point tenderness
- No increased temperature of right shoulder
- Crepitus to palpation (see Fig. 1.2)
- The drop test was negative (see Fig. 1.4)

OTHER FINDINGS OF NOTE

- Slightly elevated BP
- Normal HEENT examination
- Normal cardiovascular examination

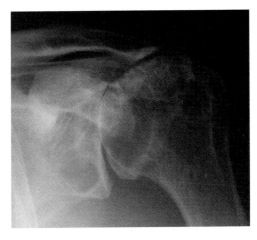

Fig. 1.5 Anteroposterior (AP) radiograph of a patient with severe glenohumeral joint osteoarthritis. Note the superior migration of the humeral head with complete loss of the subacromial space and bony eburnation of the acromion. (From Waldman S, Campbell RSD. *Imaging of Pain*. Philadelphia, PA: Saunders; 2011 [Fig. 86.2].)

- Normal pulmonary examination
- Normal abdominal examination
- No peripheral edema
- Normal upper extremity neurologic examination, motor and sensory examination
- Examination of other joints normal

 ## What Tests Would You Like to Order?

The following test was ordered:
- Plain radiographs of the right shoulder

TEST RESULTS

The plain radiographs of the right shoulder revealed severe osteoarthritis of the glenohumeral joint with loss of the subacromial space and bony eburnation of the acromium (Fig. 1.5).

 ## Clinical Correlation—Putting It All Together

What is the diagnosis?
- Osteoarthritis of the right glenohumeral joint

The Science Behind the Diagnosis

ANATOMY OF THE JOINTS OF THE SHOULDER

The shoulder is a unique joint for a variety of reasons. Unlike the knee and the hip with their inherent primary stability that results from their solid bony architecture, the shoulder is a relatively unstable joint held together by a complex combination of ligaments, tendons, muscles, and unique soft tissues—most notably, the labrum and rotator cuff. What the shoulder lacks in stability, it more than makes up for in its extensive range of motion. Although not a true weight-bearing joint like the hip or knee, the shoulder joint is subjected to extreme mechanical forces due to its extensive range of motion. Common activities such as lifting objects overhead or throwing serve to magnify these mechanical load factors and make the joint susceptible to repetitive motion injuries.

To make the most of the information gleaned from the physical examination of the shoulder, one must fully understand its functional anatomy. To fully understand the functional anatomy of the shoulder, one must recognize that the shoulder joint cannot be thought of as a single joint like the knee but rather as

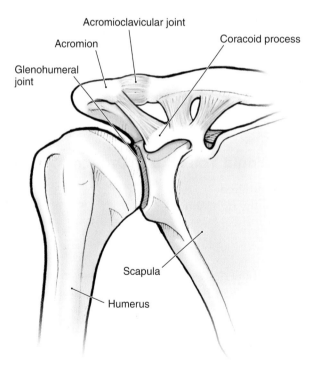

Fig. 1.6 The shoulder joint. (From Waldman S. *Pain Review*. 1st ed. Philadelphia, PA: Saunders; 2009 [Fig. 37.1].)

four separate joints working in concert to function as one (Fig. 1.6). These four joints are as follows:

- Sternoclavicular joint
- Acromioclavicular joint
- Glenohumeral joint
- Scapulothoracic joint

While the glenohumeral joint is responsible for the main functional mobility of the shoulder joint, each of the other joints works synergistically with its counterparts to allow for the extensive and extremely varied range of motion of the shoulder joint. This unique range of motion of the shoulder joint is further enhanced by the unusual physical characteristics of the humeral head and the glenoid fossa. While the articular surfaces of most joints are well matched in terms of their complementary shape with one another (e.g., the acetabulum and the femoral head), the large, rounded humeral head is amazingly mismatched to the much smaller and shallower, ovoid-shaped glenoid fossa. While this mismatch allows for the unique range of motion of the shoulder joint, it also contributes to the relative instability of the joint and is in large part responsible for the shoulder joint's propensity for injury. To this end, the shoulder joint is the most commonly dislocated large joint in the body.

CLINICAL PRESENTATION OF ARTHRITIS OF THE GLENOHUMERAL JOINT

The shoulder joint is susceptible to the development of arthritis from various conditions that cause damage to the joint cartilage (Table 1.1). Osteoarthritis is the most common cause of shoulder pain and functional disability. It may occur after seemingly minor trauma or may be the result of repeated microtrauma. Pain around the shoulder and upper arm that is worse with activity is present in most patients suffering from osteoarthritis of the shoulder. Difficulty sleeping is also common, as is progressive loss of motion.

Most patients presenting with shoulder pain secondary to osteoarthritis, rotator cuff arthropathy, or posttraumatic arthritis complain of pain that is localized around the shoulder and upper arm. Activity makes the pain worse, whereas rest and heat provide some relief. The pain is constant and is characterized as aching; it may interfere with sleep. Some patients complain of a grating or popping sensation with use of the joint, and crepitus may be present on physical examination.

In addition to pain, patients suffering from arthritis of the shoulder joint often experience a gradual reduction in functional ability because of decreasing shoulder range of motion. This change makes simple everyday tasks such as combing one's hair, fastening a brassiere, or reaching overhead quite difficult. With continued disuse, muscle wasting may occur, and a frozen shoulder may develop.

TABLE 1.1 ■ Causes of Shoulder Pain

Localized Bony or Joint Space Pathology	Periarticular Pathology	Systemic Disease	Sympathetically Mediated Pain	Referred From Other Body Areas
Fracture	Bursitis	Rheumatoid arthritis	Causalgia	Brachial plexopathy
Primary bone tumor	Tendinitis	Collagen vascular disease	Reflex sympathetic dystrophy	Cervical radiculopathy
Primary synovial tissue tumor	Rotator cuff tear	Reiter syndrome	Shoulder-hand syndrome	Cervical spondylosis
Joint instability	Impingement syndromes	Gout	Dressler syndrome	Fibromyalgia
Localized arthritis	Adhesive capsulitis	Other crystal arthropathies	Postmyocardial infarction adhesive capsulitis of the shoulder	Myofascial pain syndromes such as scapulocostal syndrome
Osteophyte formation	Joint instability	Charcot neuropathic arthritis		Parsonage-Turner syndrome (idiopathic brachial neuritis)
Joint space infection	Muscle strain			Thoracic outlet syndrome
Hemarthrosis	Periarticular infection not involving joint space			Entrapment neuropathies
Villonodular synovitis	Muscle sprain			Intrathoracic tumors
Intraarticular foreign body				Pneumothorax
				Subdiaphragmatic pathology such as subcapsular hematoma of the spleen with Kerr sign

From Waldman S. *Physical Diagnosis of Pain: An Atlas of Signs and Symptoms.* 3rd ed. St Louis, MO: Elsevier; 2016 [Table 24.1].

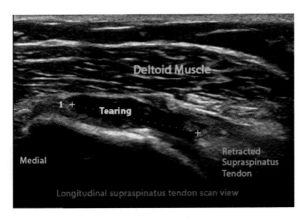

Fig. 1.7 Longitudinal ultrasound image of the shoulder demonstrating a large tear of the supraspinatus muscle. (Image credit: Steven Waldman, MD.)

TESTING

Plain radiographs are indicated in all patients who present with shoulder pain (see Fig. 1.5). Based on the patient's clinical presentation, additional testing may be indicated, including a complete blood count, erythrocyte sedimentation rate, and antinuclear antibody testing. Computerized tomography may help identify bony abnormalities. Magnetic resonance and ultrasound imaging of the shoulder are indicated if a rotator cuff tear or other soft tissue pathology is suspected (Figs. 1.7 and 1.8). Radionuclide bone scanning is indicated if metastatic disease or primary tumor involving the shoulder is a possibility (Fig. 1.9).

DIFFERENTIAL DIAGNOSIS

Osteoarthritis of the joint is the most common form of arthritis that results in shoulder pain; however, rheumatoid arthritis, posttraumatic arthritis, and rotator cuff arthropathy are also common causes of shoulder pain (Table 1.2; Fig. 1.10). Less common causes of arthritis-induced shoulder pain include collagen vascular diseases, infection, villonodular synovitis, and Lyme disease. Acute infectious arthritis is usually accompanied by significant systemic symptoms, including fever and malaise, and should be easily recognized; it is diagnosed with culture and treated with antibiotics rather than injection therapy. Collagen vascular diseases generally manifest as a polyarthropathy rather than a monoarthropathy limited to the shoulder joint; however, shoulder pain secondary to collagen vascular disease responds exceedingly well to the intraarticular injection technique described here.

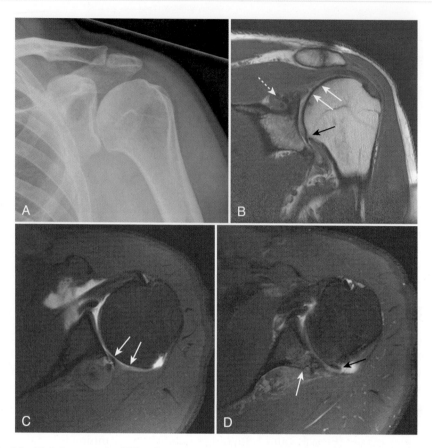

Fig. 1.8 (A) Anteroposterior (AP) radiograph of a patient with early osteoarthritis (OA) of the gleno-humeral joint. There is asymmetric joint space narrowing and minor inferior osteophyte formation. The acromioclavicular (AC) joint is normal, and the subacromial space is preserved. (B) The coronal T1-weighted (T1W) magnetic resonance (MR) arthrogram image demonstrates chondral thinning *(white arrows)*, the inferior osteophyte *(black arrow)*, and low—signal intensity (SI) loose bodies within the spinoglenoid notch *(broken arrow)*. (C) The chondral thinning is also seen on an axial T1W with fat suppression (FST1W) MR image *(white arrows)*. (D) On a more inferior axial FST1W MR image, the osteophytes *(black arrow)* are visualized in association with bony eburnation of the posterior glenoid *(thick white arrow)*. (From Waldman SD, Campbell RSD. *Imaging of Pain*. Philadelphia, PA: Saunders; 2011 [Fig. 86.1].)

TREATMENT

Initial treatment of the pain and functional disability associated with osteoarthritis of the shoulder includes a combination of nonsteroidal antiinflammatory drugs (NSAIDs) or cyclooxygenase-2 (COX-2) inhibitors and physical therapy. Local application of heat and cold may also be beneficial, as may be the topical application of capsaicin. For patients who do not respond to these treatment

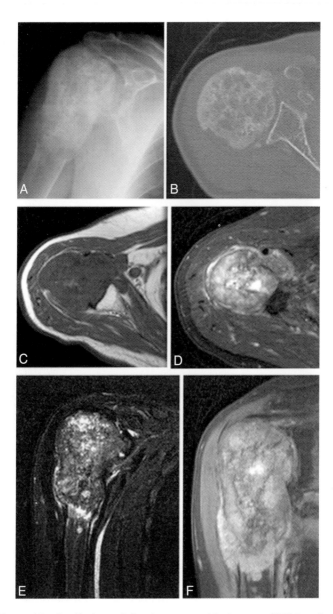

Fig. 1.9 A 67-year-old male with clear-cell chondrosarcoma of the humerus. (A) Plain radiograph of proximal right humerus demonstrates diffuse sclerosis. Also evident are articular margins, irregularities reconstituted by tumor matrix, ill-defined glenoid, and increase in matrix density in the subcoracoid bursal space. (B) Axial computed tomography (CT) of proximal humerus at tip of coracoids demonstrates intraarticular bodies and tumor matrix in the medullary canal with disorganized cortical margination and reactive sclerosis. (C, D) Comparable axial T1 and T2 with fat saturation at inferior glenoid. Note complete fat marrow replacement and extension of tumor into anteromedial joint recess and expansion of lesser tuberosity. (E) Coronal inversion recovery demonstrates diffuse marrow involvement and tumor involving the articular segment and extending into the metadiaphyseal junction with permeation of the cortices and medial subcoracoid extension into the joint. (F) Postgadolinium imaging shows heterogeneous enhancing tumor, replacement of marrow cavity cortices, and periosteal surface with extension along undersurface of the supraspinatus tendon of the rotator cuff and diaphyseal satellite lesions. (From Elojeimy S, Ahrens WA, Howard B, et al. Clear-cell chondrosarcoma of the humerus. *Radiol Case Rep.* 2013;8(2):848 [Fig. 1].)

TABLE 1.2 ■ Differential Diagnosis of Shoulder Pain *(Continued)*

Diagnosis	Age	Type of Onset	Location of Pain	Night Pain	Active Range of Motion	Passive Range of Motion
Rotator cuff tendinitis	Any	Acute or chronic	Deltoid region	+	↓↓ Guarding	Normal
Rotator cuff tears (chronic)	Older than 40 years	Often chronic	Deltoid region	++	↓↓	Normal (may later ↓)
Bicipital tendinitis	Any	Overuse	Anterior	− −	↓ Guarding	Normal
Calcific tendinitis	30–60 years old	Acute	Point of shoulder	++	↓↓ Guarding	Normal except for pain
Capsulitis ("frozen shoulder")	Older than 40 years	Insidious	Deep in shoulder	++	↓↓	↓↓
Acromio-clavicular joint	Any	Acute or chronic	Over joint	Lying on side	↓ Full elevation	Normal
Osteoarthrosis of gleno-humeral joint	Older than 40 years usually	Insidious	Deep in shoulder	++	↓↓	↓↓
Glenohumeral instability	25 years	Episodic	Anterior or posterior	− −	Only apprehension	Only apprehension
Cervical spondylosis	Older than 40 years	Insidious	Suprascapular	Often	Normal	Normal
Thoracic outlet syndrome	Any	Usually with activity	Neck, shoulder, arm	− −	Normal	Normal
Sympathetically mediated pain	Any	With contact	Neck, shoulder, arm, diffuse	Often	↓ Guarding	↓ Guarding

From Waldman S. *Physical Diagnosis of Pain: An Atlas of Signs and Symptoms*. 3rd ed. St Louis, MO: Elsevier; 2016 [Table 24.2].

modalities, intraarticular injection of local anesthetic and steroid is a reasonable next step.

Intraarticular injection of the shoulder is performed by placing the patient in the supine position and preparing the skin overlying the shoulder, subacromial region, and joint space with antiseptic solution. Using strict aseptic technique, the practitioner attaches a sterile syringe containing 2 mL of 0.25% preservative-free bupivacaine and 40 mg methylprednisolone to a 1.5-inch, 25-gauge needle. The midpoint of the acromion is identified, and at a point approximately 1 inch below the midpoint, the shoulder joint space is identified

Impingement Signs	Radiation of Pain	Paresthesia	Weakness	Instability	Radiographic Changes	Special Features
+ + +	– –	– –	Only due to pain	Look for	In chronic cases	Painful arc of abduction
+ +	– –	– –	+ +	– –	+	Wasting of cuff muscles
+	Occasionally into biceps	– –	Only due to pain	Look for	None	Special examination tests
+ + +	– –	– –	Only due to pain	– –	+ +	Tenderness+ +
+	– –	– –	– –	– –	– –	Global range of motion ↓
– –	– –	– –	– –	– –	In chronic cases	Local tenderness
– –	– –	– –	May have mild + with acute episodes	– –	+ + +	Crepitus
Possible	– –	+ With acute episodes	+ + +	Often	Stress tests	
– –	+ +	+ + +	+	– –	In cervical spine	Pain with neck movement
– –	+ +	+ +	+ +	– –	– –	Special examination tests
Possible	Ill defined	– –	With disuse	– –	+ Bone scan, articular changes, and demineralization	Vasomotor and sudomotor changes

(Fig. 1.11). The needle is carefully advanced through the skin and subcutaneous tissues, through the joint capsule, and into the joint. If bone is encountered, the needle is withdrawn into the subcutaneous tissues and is redirected superiorly and slightly more medially. After the joint space is entered, the contents of the syringe are gently injected. Little resistance to injection is felt; if resistance is encountered, the needle is probably in a ligament or tendon and should be advanced slightly into the joint space until the injection can proceed without significant resistance. The needle is then removed, and a sterile pressure dressing and ice pack are applied to the injection site. Recent clinical

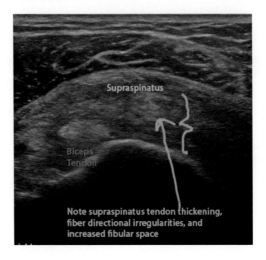

Fig. 1.10   Ultrasound image demonstrating rotator cuff tendinopathy. (Image credit: Steven Waldman, MD)

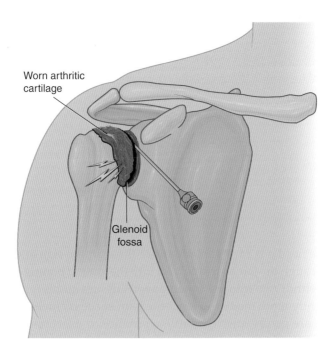

Fig. 1.11   Intraarticular injection of the glenohumeral joint. (From Waldman SD. *Atlas of Pain Management Injection Techniques*. 4th ed. St Louis, MO: Elsevier; 2017 [Fig. 26.2].)

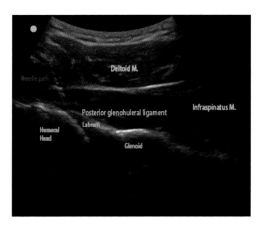

Fig. 1.12 Ultrasound guided intraarticular injection of the glenohumeral joint. (Image credit: Steven Waldman, MD)

experience has suggested that the injection of platelet-rich plasma into the glenohumeral joint may provide improvement of the pain and functional disability associated with osteoarthritis of the shoulder. Ultrasound needle guidance may aid in the intraarticular placement of the needle in patients in whom anatomic landmarks are difficult to identify (Fig. 1.12).

Physical modalities, including local heat and gentle range of motion exercises, should be introduced several days after the patient undergoes injection for shoulder pain. Vigorous exercises should be avoided because they will exacerbate the patient's symptoms.

HIGH-YIELD TAKEAWAYS

- The patient is afebrile, making an acute infectious etiology (e.g., septic arthritis) unlikely.
- The patient's symptomatology is not the result of acute trauma but more likely the result of repetitive microtrauma that has damaged the joint over time.
- The patient's pain is diffuse rather than highly localized as would be the case with a pathologic process like subdeltoid bursitis.
- The patient's symptoms are unilateral and only involve one joint, which is more suggestive of a local process than a systemic polyarthropathy.
- Sleep disturbance is common and must be addressed concurrently with the patient's pain symptomatology.
- Plain radiographs will provide high-yield information regarding the bony contents of the joint, but ultrasound imaging and magnetic resonance imaging will be more useful in identifying soft tissue pathology.

Suggested Readings

Allen H, Chan BY, Davis KW, et al. Overuse injuries of the shoulder. *Radiol Clin N Am.* 2019;57(5):897—909.

Cibulas A, Leyva A, Cibulas G, et al. Acute shoulder injury. *Radiol Clin N Am.* 2019;57 (5):883—896.

Netter FH. Shoulder (glenohumeral joint). In: *Atlas of Human Anatomy.* 4th ed. Philadelphia, PA: Saunders; 2006.

Reschke D, Dagrosa R, Matteson DT. An unusual cause of shoulder pain and weakness. *Am J Emerg Med.* 2018;36(12):2339.e5—2339.e6.

Waldman SD. Clinical correlates: functional anatomy of the shoulder. In: *Physical Diagnosis of Pain: An Atlas of Signs and Symptoms.* 3rd ed. Philadelphia, PA: Saunders; 2016.

Waldman SD. Rotator cuff tear. In: *Atlas of Common Pain Syndromes.* 4th ed. Philadelphia, PA: Elsevier; 2019:129—133.

Terrell Williams

A 28-Year-Old Male With Left Shoulder Pain

- Learn the common causes of shoulder pain.
- Develop an understanding of the unique anatomy of the shoulder joint.
- Develop an understanding of the causes of acromioclavicular joint pain.
- Develop an understanding of the various types of acromioclavicular joint injury.
- Learn the clinical presentation of osteoarthritis of the acromioclavicular joint.
- Learn how to examine the shoulder.
- Learn how to use physical examination to identify pathology of the acromioclavicular joint.
- Develop an understanding of the treatment options for acromioclavicular joint pain.

Terrell Williams

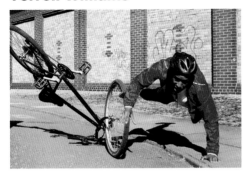

Terrell Williams is a 28-year-old bicycle messenger with the chief complaint of "my left shoulder is killing me." Terrell stated that about a week ago, a kid threw a rock at him while he was delivering some papers for a lawyer on his route. "The rock flew out of nowhere and it startled me. The next thing I knew I was falling. I put out my left hand to try and break my fall, but I landed really hard anyway." I asked if he was wearing a helmet and he gave me the "are you kidding me" look as he answered that he always wears a helmet. "Good," I said, then asked, "So did you hit your head?" He said, "No, but I really banged up the palm of my left hand and had to dig out some gravel and splinters."

I asked Terrell if he had anything like this happen before. He shook his head and responded, "Never. I saw the kid out of the corner of my eye, but things just happened too fast." "What I meant, Terrell, was have you ever passed out or lost concentration and fallen off your bike?" "No, that has never happened. I am very careful with all the distracted driving and all. You know what I mean? What worries me is that my left shoulder isn't working right and it is making it hard to ride. It feels like something has come loose inside the joint. I am even having a hard time getting my coffee cup off the cupboard shelf."

I asked Terrell about any antecedent shoulder trauma and he just shook his head no. "Doc, I was never much for sports, but I love my bike. I tried some Advil and Tylenol and they don't do much." I asked Terrell what made his pain worse and he said, "Anytime I use my left shoulder, it hurts." Terrell went on to say that when he reached up, he felt a kind of grating sensation, especially in the morning when he first got up. I asked how he was sleeping and he shook his head and said, "Doc, I'll bet this shoulder wakes me up one hundred times a night. I usually sleep on my left side, but since I fell, I can't do that, so I try to sleep on my right side. Every time I roll over to my left side, my shoulder wakes me up."

I asked Terrell to point with one finger to show me where it hurts the most. He pointed to the anterior aspect of the shoulder and said, "Doc, it's right here where something is wrong. It feels like something is loose in there and the whole shoulder feels kind of squishy or swollen up." I asked if he had any fever or chills and he shook his head no.

On physical examination, Terrell was afebrile. His respirations were 16 and his pulse was 68 and regular. His blood pressure (BP) was 112/70. His head,

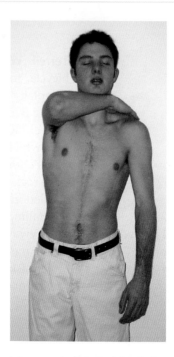

Fig. 2.1 The chin adduction test for acromioclavicular joint dysfunction is performed by having the patient abduct the affected arm to 90 degrees. The patient is then instructed to adduct the affected arm and shoulder directly under the chin and grasp the contralateral shoulder. Patients who suffer from acromioclavicular joint dysfunction will experience a marked increase in pain with adduction. (From Waldman SD. *Physical Diagnosis of Pain: An Atlas of Signs and Symptoms*. 3rd ed. St Louis, MO: Elsevier; 2016 [Fig. 62.1].)

eyes, ears, nose, throat (HEENT) exam was normal, as was his cardiopulmonary examination. His thyroid was normal. His abdominal examination revealed no abnormal mass or organomegaly. There was no costovertebral angle (CVA) tenderness. There was no peripheral edema. His low back examination was unremarkable. Visual inspection of the left shoulder revealed a small area of resolving ecchymosis anteriorly. I noted that Terrell was splinting his left shoulder by holding his left upper extremity close to his side. The shoulder was a little warm, but did not appear to be infected. The left shoulder felt slightly edematous on palpation, but there was no point tenderness over the deltoid. Palpation of the acromioclavicular joint exacerbated Terrell's pain. I did not appreciate any obvious separation of the joint. I performed a cross-body adduction test and an adduction stress test, which were both positive on the left and negative on the right (Figs. 2.1 and 2.2). The right shoulder examination was normal, as was examination of his other major joints. A careful neurologic examination of the

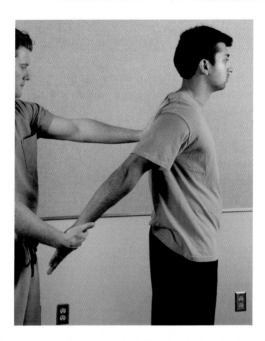

Fig. 2.2 The adduction stress test for acromioclavicular joint dysfunction is performed by having the patient maximally extend the affected shoulder and arm behind him or her while the examiner exerts forward pressure on the scapula. (From Waldman SD. *Physical Diagnosis of Pain: An Atlas of Signs and Symptoms*. 3rd ed. St Louis, MO: Elsevier; 2016 [Fig. 61.6].)

upper extremities revealed that there was no evidence of peripheral or entrapment neuropathy, and the deep tendon reflexes were normal.

Key Clinical Points—What's Important and What's Not

THE HISTORY

- A history of acute trauma
- A history of falling onto an outstretched hand
- No history of previous significant shoulder pain
- No fever of chills
- Acute onset of shoulder pain following traumatic event with exacerbation of pain with shoulder use
- Grinding sensation in the right shoulder
- Sleep disturbance
- Difficulty elevating the affected upper extremity

THE PHYSICAL EXAMINATION

- The patient is afebrile
- Resolving echymosis present over anterior shoulder on the left
- Palpation of right shoulder reveals tenderness anteriorly
- The shoulder is slightly swollen
- No evidence of infection
- Crepitus to palpation
- The chin adduction test was positive (see Fig. 2.1)
- The adduction stress test was positive (see Fig. 2.2)

OTHER FINDINGS OF NOTE

- Normal HEENT examination
- Normal cardiovascular examination
- Normal pulmonary examination
- Normal abdominal examination
- No peripheral edema
- Normal upper extremity motor and sensory examination
- Examination of other joints was normal

What Tests Would You Like to Order?

The following tests were ordered:
- Plain radiographs of the left shoulder, including anteroposterior [AP], lateral, and axillary views
- Plain radiograph of the scapula, including a lateral scapular view

TEST RESULTS

The plain radiographs of the left shoulder revealed no evidence of acromioclavicular separation with normal coracoclavicular and acromioclavicular distances (Fig. 2.3). The radiograph of the scapula revealed no fracture or other abnormality.

Clinical Correlation—Putting It All Together

What is the diagnosis?
- Acromioclavicular joint pain secondary to acute traumatic injury

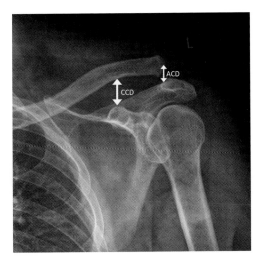

Fig. 2.3 Normal radiograph of the acromioclavicular joint with normal coracoclavicular distance *(CCD)* and acromioclavicular distance *(ACD)*. (From Horst C, Garving T, Thometzki P, et al. Comparative study on the treatment of Rockwood type III acute acromioclavicular dislocation: clinical results from the TightRope® technique vs. K-wire fixation. *OTSR.* 2017;103(2):171–176.)

The Science Behind the Diagnosis

ANATOMY OF THE ACROMIOCLAVICULAR JOINT

The acromioclavicular joint is formed by the distal end of the clavicle and the anterior and medial aspects of the acromion (Fig. 2.4). The strength of the joint arises in large part from the dense coracoclavicular ligament, which attaches the bottom of the distal end of the clavicle to the coracoid process. A small indentation can be felt where the clavicle abuts the acromion. The joint is completely surrounded by an articular capsule. The superior portion of the joint is covered by the superior acromioclavicular ligament, which attaches the distal clavicle to the upper surface of the acromion. The inferior portion of the joint is covered by the inferior acromioclavicular ligament, which attaches the inferior portion of the distal clavicle to the acromion. Both of these ligaments further add to the joint's stability. The acromioclavicular joint may or may not contain an articular disk. The volume of the acromioclavicular joint space is small, and care must be taken not to disrupt the joint by forcefully injecting large volumes of local anesthetic and corticosteroid into the intraarticular space when performing this injection technique.

CLINICAL CONSIDERATIONS

The acromioclavicular joint is vulnerable to injury from both acute trauma and repetitive microtrauma. Acute injuries frequently take the form of falls directly

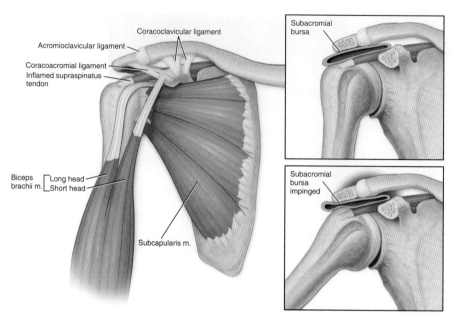

Fig. 2.4 The anatomy of the acromioclavicular joint. (From Waldman SD. Subacromial impingement syndrome. In: Waldman SD, ed. *Atlas of Uncommon Pain Syndromes*. 3rd ed. Philadelphia, PA: Saunders; 2014 [Fig. 30.2].)

onto the shoulder when playing sports or falling from a bicycle. Repeated strain from throwing injuries or working with the arm raised across the body also may result in trauma to the joint. After trauma, the joint may become acutely inflamed; if the condition becomes chronic, arthritis of the acromioclavicular joint may develop.

The patient with acromioclavicular joint pain frequently reports increased pain when reaching across the chest. Often the patient is unable to sleep on the affected shoulder and may report a grinding sensation in the joint, especially on first awakening. Physical examination may reveal enlargement or swelling of the joint with tenderness to palpation. Downward traction or passive adduction of the affected shoulder may cause increased pain. The chin adduction test will also help confirm the diagnosis. This test is performed by having the patient abduct the affected arm to 90 degrees and then adduct the arm across the chest just under the chin with the objective of grasping the contralateral shoulder (see Fig. 2.1). Patients with acromioclavicular joint dysfunction will experience severe pain and often will be unable to repeat the maneuver. Furthermore, if there is disruption of the ligaments of the acromioclavicular joint, these maneuvers may reveal joint instability.

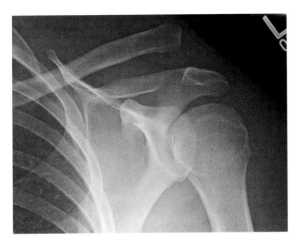

Fig. 2.5 A 32-year-old male with type III acromioclavicular joint (ACJ) dislocation. Anteroposterior (AP) radiograph shows superior dislocation of distal clavicle from ACJ, with increased coracoclavicular interval, indicating disruption of coracoclavicular ligaments of the lesion. (From Bindra J, VanDenBogaerde J, Hunter JC. Coracoid fracture with recurrent AC joint separation after tightrope repair of AC joint dislocation. *Radiol Case Rep*. 2011;6(4):624.)

TABLE 2.1 ■ Radiographic Classification of Injuries of the Acromioclavicular Joint

- Type I: Normal
- Type II: Subluxation of the acromioclavicular joint space is less than 1 cm; normal coracoclavicular space
- Type III: Subluxation of the acromioclavicular joint space is greater than 1 cm; widening of the coraco-clavicular space is more than 50%
- Types IV–VI: Subluxation of the acromioclavicular joint space is more than 1 cm and widening of the coracoclavicular space is more than 50%; there is associated displacement of the clavicle

TESTING

Plain radiographs are indicated in all patients who present with acute shoulder pain following traumatic injury (see Fig. 2.3). If acromioclavicular joint injury is suspected, AP, lateral, and axillary views of the shoulder should be obtained as well as a lateral radiograph of the scapula (Fig. 2.5). Radiographic findings may help characterize the extent of ligamentous injury (Table 2.1). Based on the patient's clinical presentation, additional testing may be indicated, including a complete blood count, erythrocyte sedimentation rate, and antinuclear antibody testing. Computerized tomography may help identify bony abnormalities, including septic arthritis (Fig. 2.6). Magnetic resonance (MRI) and ultrasound imaging of the

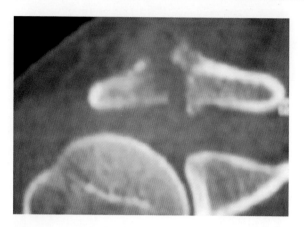

Fig. 2.6 Computed tomography of the right shoulder showing erosions on both sides of the acromio-clavicular joint, consistent with septic arthritis. (From Bossert M, Prati C, Bertolini E, et al. Septic arthritis of the acromioclavicular joint. *Joint Bone Spine*. 2010;77(5):466–469.)

shoulder is indicated if disruption of the acromioclavicular ligaments is suspected (Figs. 2.7 and 2.8). Radionuclide bone scanning is indicated if metastatic disease or primary tumor involving the shoulder is a possibility.

DIFFERENTIAL DIAGNOSIS

In the presence of trauma, the focus of the evaluation is to identify ligamentous injury and fractures, especially of the acromion and coronoid. Occult scapular fractures can be easily missed, so a high index of suspicion is indicated. In the absence of trauma, osteoarthritis of the acromioclavicular joint is the most common form of arthritis that results in shoulder pain; however, rheumatoid arthritis, posttraumatic arthritis, and rotator cuff arthropathy are also common causes of shoulder pain (Table 2.2, Fig. 2.9). Less common causes of arthritis-induced shoulder pain include collagen vascular diseases, infection, brachial plexopathies, and Lyme disease. Acute infectious arthritis is usually accompanied by significant systemic symptoms, including fever and malaise, and should be easily recognized; it is diagnosed with culture and treated with antibiotics rather than injection therapy. Collagen vascular diseases generally manifest as a polyarthropathy rather than a monoarthropathy limited to the shoulder joint; however, shoulder pain secondary to collagen vascular disease responds exceedingly well to the intraarticular injection technique described here.

TREATMENT

Initial treatment of the pain and functional disability associated with osteoarthritis of the shoulder includes a combination of nonsteroidal antiinflammatory

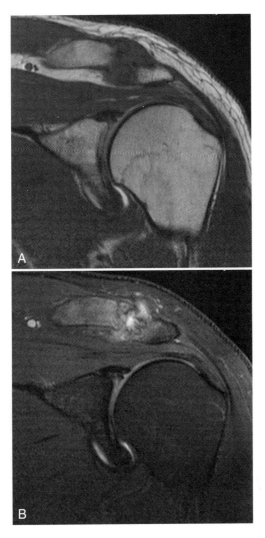

Fig. 2.7 (A) Magnetic resonance imaging of the acromioclavicular joint demonstrating osteoarthritis with marrow edema and subchondral cyst formation. (B) Subluxation of the acromioclavicular joint is also noted indicating joint instability. (From Waldman SD, Campbell R. *Imaging of Pain*. Philadelphia, PA: Saunders; 2011 [Fig. 89.3].)

drugs (NSAIDs) or cyclooxygenase-2 (COX-2) inhibitors and physical therapy. Local application of heat and cold may also be beneficial, as may be the topical application of capsaicin. For patients who do not respond to these treatment modalities, intraarticular injection of local anesthetic and steroid is a reasonable next step.

Intraarticular injection of the acromioclavicular joint is performed by placing the patient in the supine position and preparing the skin overlying the joint space

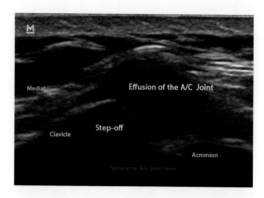

Fig. 2.8 Transverse ultrasound imaging of the acromioclavicular joint revealing an effusion and a small stepoff suggestive of ligamentous injury. (Courtesy Steven Waldman, MD.)

TABLE 2.2 ■ Differential Diagnosis of Acromioclavicular Joint Pain

- Clavicle fractures
- Coracoid fractures
- Rotator cuff injury
- Shoulder dislocation
- Shoulder impingement syndrome
- Osteoarthritis
- Inflammatory arthritis
- Glenoid labrum tear
- Septic arthritis
- Brachial plexus injury
- Parsonage-Turner syndrome
- Os acrominale
- Distal clavicle osteolysis

From Waldman SD. *Physical Diagnosis of Pain: An Atlas of Signs and Symptoms*. 3rd ed. St Louis, MO: Elsevier; 2016 [Table 24.2].

with antiseptic solution. With strict aseptic technique, the tip of the acromion is identified, and at a point approximately 1 inch medially, the acromioclavicular joint space is identified. The needle is then carefully advanced through the skin and subcutaneous tissues medially at a 20-degree angle through the joint capsule into the joint (Fig. 2.10). If bone is encountered, the needle is withdrawn into the subcutaneous tissues and redirected slightly more medially. After the joint space has been entered, the contents of the syringe are gently injected. There should be some resistance to injection, because the joint space is small and the joint capsule is dense. If significant resistance is encountered, the needle is probably in a ligament and should be advanced or withdrawn slightly into the joint space until the injection proceeds with only limited resistance. If no resistance is encountered on

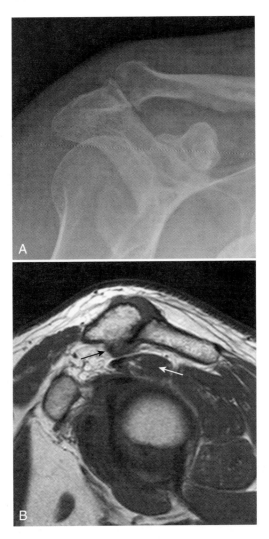

Fig. 2.9 (A) Oblique radiograph of the acromioclavicular joint demonstrating osteophytes and bony sclerosis consistent with osteoarthritis. (B) Sagittal oblique T1-weighted magnetic resonance imaging shows inferior osteophyte formation. (From Waldman SD, Campbell RSD. *Imaging of Pain*. Philadelphia, PA: Saunders; 2011 [Fig. 89.1].)

injection, the joint capsule is probably not intact and arthrography and/or MRI of the joint is recommended. The needle is then removed and a sterile pressure dressing and ice pack are placed at the injection site.

Ultrasound needle guidance may aid in the intraarticular placement of the needle in patients in whom anatomic landmarks are difficult to identify (Fig. 2.11).

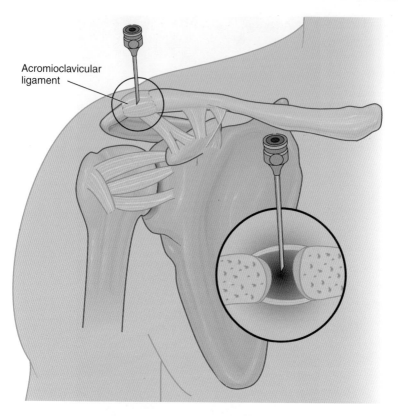

Acromioclavicular
ligament

Fig. 2.10 Acromioclavicular joint injection technique. (From Waldman SD. *Atlas of Pain Management Injection Techniques*. 4th ed. St Louis, MO: Elsevier; 2017 [Fig. 27.4].)

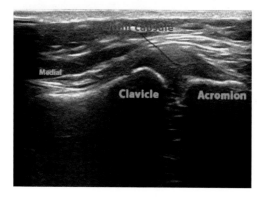

Fig. 2.11 Anatomy for ultrasound-guided injection of the acromioclavicular joint. (Courtesy Steven Waldman, MD.)

Physical modalities, including local heat and gentle range of motion exercises, should be introduced several days after the patient undergoes injection for shoulder pain. Vigorous exercises should be avoided because they will exacerbate the patient's symptoms.

HIGH-YIELD TAKEAWAYS

- The patient is afebrile, making an acute infectious etiology (e.g., septic arthritis) unlikely.
- The patient's symptomatology is the result of acute trauma, and physical examination and testing should be focused on the identification of ligamentous injury and fracture.
- The patient's pain is localized to the acromioclavicular joint.
- The patient's symptoms are unilateral and only involve one joint, which is more suggestive of a local process than a systemic polyarthropathy.
- Sleep disturbance is common and must be addressed concurrently with the patient's pain symptomatology.
- Plain radiographs will provide high-yield information regarding the bony contents of the joint, but ultrasound imaging and MRI will be more useful in identifying soft tissue pathology.

Suggested Readings

Allen H, Chan BY, Davis KW, et al. Overuse injuries of the shoulder. *Radiol Clin N Am.* 2019;57(5):897–909.

Cibulas A, Leyva A, Cibulas G, et al. Acute shoulder injury. *Radiol Clin N Am.* 2019;57(5):883–896.

Netter FH. Shoulder (glenohumeral joint). In: *Atlas of Human Anatomy.* 4th ed. Philadelphia PA: Saunders; 2006.

Reschke D, Dagrosa R, Matteson DT. An unusual cause of shoulder pain and weakness. *Am J Emerg Med.* 2018;36(12):2339.e5–2339.e6.

Waldman SD. Clinical correlates: functional anatomy of the shoulder. In: *Physical Diagnosis of Pain: An Atlas of Signs and Symptoms.* 3rd ed. Philadelphia PA: Saunders; 2016.

Rotator cuff tear. In: Waldman SD, ed. *Atlas of Common Pain Syndromes.* 4th ed. Philadelphia, PA: Elsevier; 2019:129–133.

Daisy Chang

A 26-Year-Old Female With Severe Left Shoulder Pain With Associated Swelling

LEARNING OBJECTIVES

- Learn the common causes of shoulder pain.
- Develop an understanding of the unique anatomy of the shoulder joint.
- Develop an understanding of the bursae of the shoulder.
- Develop an understanding of the causes of subdeltoid bursitis.
- Develop an understanding of the differential diagnosis of subdeltoid bursitis.
- Learn the clinical presentation of subdeltoid bursitis.
- Learn how to examine the shoulder.
- Learn how to use physical examination to identify subdeltoid bursitis.
- Develop an understanding of the treatment options for subdeltoid bursitis.

Daisy Chang

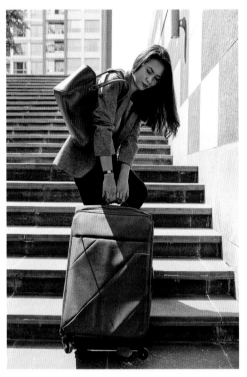

Daisy Chang is a 27-year-old pharmaceutical representative with the chief complaint of "my left shoulder is killing me." Daisy stated that she was traveling to a medical meeting in Montreal about a 3 week ago when she did something "really stupid." Daisy went on to say that she decided to take the train up to Montreal from New York so she could get some work done while on the train. When she went to get an Uber to take her to her hotel, she saw that prices were surging, so she decided to walk. "I had on pretty good shoes and I wanted to get my steps in after sitting on the train, but I didn't understand that there were about 100 flights of stairs between me and the hotel. As usual, I had overpacked and my rolly bag was really heavy, but, I thought, no big deal, and off I went. It really wasn't that far of a walk to the hotel, but dragging that bag up all of those stairs really did my shoulder in. I was a real idiot!"

I asked Daisy about any antecedent shoulder trauma and she just shook her head no, but went on to say that from time to time her left shoulder would bother her a little after playing golf, but a couple of Advil and she was good to go. This time, the pain just wouldn't go away in spite of using the Advil and a heating pad. Daisy said that she felt that her shoulder was kind of swollen and "squishy" and that it felt hot to touch. I asked Daisy what made her pain worse and she said, "Anytime I lift my left arm, I feel a sudden sharp pain and a kind of catching sensation. It really hurts and the pain is messing with my sleep. Every time I roll over onto my left side, the pain in my left shoulder wakes me up."

I asked Daisy to point with one finger where it hurt the most. She pointed to the lateral aspect of the left shoulder and said, "Doctor, it's really the whole shoulder that hurts," and she cupped her left shoulder in her right palm to emphasize the point.

On physical examination, Daisy was afebrile. Her respirations were 18, and her pulse was 64 and regular. Her blood pressure (BP) was 119/68. Daisy's HEENT (head, eyes, ears, nose, throat) exam was normal, as was her cardiopulmonary examination. Her thyroid was normal. Her abdominal examination revealed no abnormal mass or organomegaly. There was no costovertebral angle (CVA) tenderness. There was no peripheral edema. Her low back examination was unremarkable. Visual inspection of the left shoulder revealed some swelling. I noted that Daisy was splinting her left shoulder by holding her left upper extremity close to her side. The shoulder was warm, but did not appear to be infected. The left shoulder felt edematous on palpation, and there was marked point tenderness over the deltoid. Palpation of the deltoid muscle exacerbated Daisy's pain. Range of motion of the glenohumeral joint, especially abduction of the joint, caused Daisy to cry out in pain. A drop arm test was positive on the left and negative on the right (Fig. 3.1). The right shoulder examination was normal, as was examination of her other major joints. A careful neurologic examination of the upper extremities revealed that there was no evidence of peripheral or entrapment neuropathy, and the deep tendon reflexes were normal.

Key Clinical Points—What's Important and What's Not

THE HISTORY

- A history of acute trauma
- No history of previous significant shoulder pain
- No fever of chills
- Acute onset of shoulder pain following traumatic event with exacerbation of pain with shoulder use
- Swelling of the left shoulder
- Sleep disturbance
- Difficulty abducting the affected upper extremity

THE PHYSICAL EXAMINATION

- The patient is afebrile
- Point tenderness to palpation of the deltoid
- Palpation of right shoulder reveals warmth to touch
- The shoulder is swollen
- No evidence of infection
- Pain on range of motion, especially abduction of the affected left shoulder
- The drop arm test was positive on the left (see Fig. 3.1)

OTHER FINDINGS OF NOTE

- Normal HEENT examination
- Normal cardiovascular examination
- Normal pulmonary examination

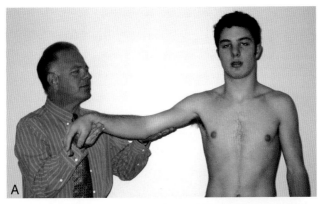

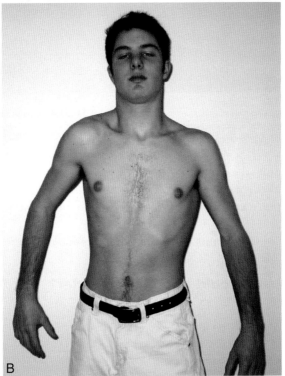

Fig. 3.1   (A) The drop arm test for subdeltoid bursitis shows the examiner supports the abducted arm. (B) The drop arm test for subdeltoid bursitis shows the abducted arm is released. (From Waldman SD. *Physical Diagnosis of Pain: An Atlas of Signs and Symptoms*. 3rd ed. St Louis, MO: Elsevier; 2016 [Figs. 59.1, 59.2].)

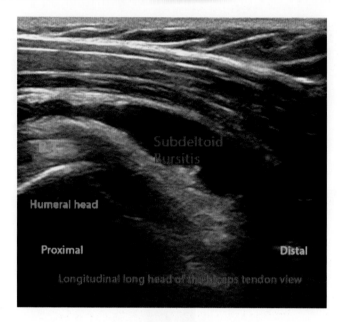

Fig. 3.2 Longitudinal ultrasound image of subdeltoid bursitis. Note relationship of the biceps tendon *(B.T.)*, the bursa, and the humeral head. (From Waldman SD. *Atlas of Common Pain Syndromes*. 4th ed. Philadelphia, PA: Elsevier; 2019 [Fig. 27.3].)

- Normal abdominal examination
- No peripheral edema
- Normal upper extremity neurologic examination, motor and sensory examination
- Examination of other joints other than the left shoulder were normal

 What Tests Would You Like to Order?

The following tests were ordered:
- Plain radiographs of the left shoulder
- Ultrasound of the left shoulder

TEST RESULTS

The plain radiographs of the left shoulder revealed soft tissue swelling and mild calcification of the subdeltoid bursa. Ultrasound examination of the left shoulder revealed an effusion around the subdeltoid bursa (Fig. 3.2).

 Clinical Correlation—Putting It All Together

What is the diagnosis?
- Subdeltoid bursitis

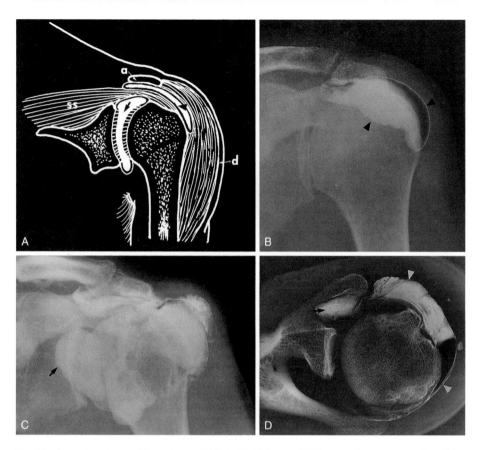

Fig. 3.3 Normal anatomy of the subacromial (subdeltoid) bursa. (A) Diagram of a coronal section of the shoulder shows the glenohumeral joint *(arrow)* and subacromial (subdeltoid) bursa *(arrowhead)*, separated by a portion of the rotator cuff (i.e., supraspinatus tendon). The supraspinatus *(ss)* and deltoid *(d)* muscles and the acromion *(a)* are indicated. (B) Subdeltoid-subacromial bursogram, accomplished with the injection of both radiopaque contrast material and air, shows the bursa *(arrowheads)* sitting like a cap on the humeral head and greater tuberosity of the humerus. Note that the joint is not opacified, indicative of an intact rotator cuff. (C) In a different cadaver, a subacromial-subdeltoid bursogram shows much more extensive structure as a result of opacification of the subacromial, subdeltoid, and subcoracoid *(arrow)* portions of the bursa. (D) Radiograph of a transverse section of the specimen illustrated in (C) shows both the subdeltoid *(arrow-heads)* and subcoracoid *(arrow)* portions of the bursa. The glenohumeral joint is not opacified. (From Waldman SD. *Atlas of Common Pain Syndromes*. 4th ed. Philadelphia, PA: Elsevier; 2019 [Fig. 27.1].)

The Science Behind the Diagnosis

ANATOMY

The subdeltoid bursa lies primarily under the acromion and extends laterally between the deltoid muscle and the joint capsule under the deltoid muscle (Fig. 3.3). It may exist as a single bursal sac or, in some patients, as a multiseg-mented series of loculated sacs.

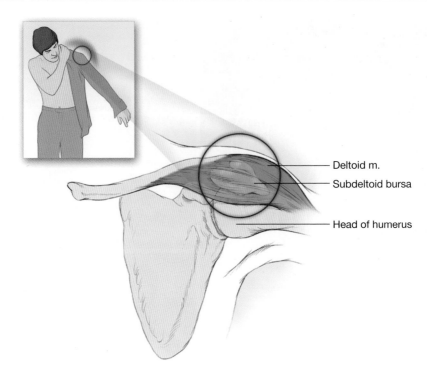

Fig. 3.4 Abduction of the shoulder exacerbates the pain of subdeltoid bursitis. (From Waldman SD. *Atlas of Common Pain Syndromes*. 4th ed. Philadelphia, PA: Elsevier; 2019 [Fig. 27.2].)

CLINICAL SYNDROME

The subdeltoid bursa is vulnerable to injury from both acute trauma and repeated microtrauma. Acute injuries frequently take the form of direct trauma to the shoulder when playing sports or falling off a bicycle. Repeated strain from throwing, bowling, carrying a heavy briefcase, working with the arm raised across the body, rotator cuff injuries, or repetitive motion associated with assembly-line work may result in inflammation of the subdeltoid bursa. If the inflammation becomes chronic, calcification of the bursa may occur.

Patients suffering from subdeltoid bursitis frequently complain of pain with any movement of the shoulder, but especially with abduction (Fig. 3.4). The pain is localized to the subdeltoid area, with referred pain often noted at the insertion of the deltoid at the deltoid tuberosity on the upper third of the humerus. Patients are often unable to sleep on the affected shoulder and may complain of a sharp, catching sensation when abducting the shoulder, especially on first awakening.

SIGNS AND SYMPTOMS

Physical examination may reveal point tenderness over the acromion; occasionally, swelling of the bursa gives the affected deltoid muscle an edematous feel. Passive elevation and medial rotation of the affected shoulder reproduce the pain, as do resisted abduction and lateral rotation. Sudden release of resistance during the maneuver markedly increases the pain. Rotator cuff tear may mimic or coexist with subdeltoid bursitis and may confuse the diagnosis.

TESTING

Plain radiographs of the shoulder may reveal calcification of the bursa and associated structures, consistent with chronic inflammation (Fig. 3.5A). Magnetic resonance imaging (MRI) is indicated if tendinitis, impingement syndromes, partial disruption of the ligaments, or rotator cuff tear is being considered (see Fig. 3.5B). Ultrasound imaging may further delineate the cause of the

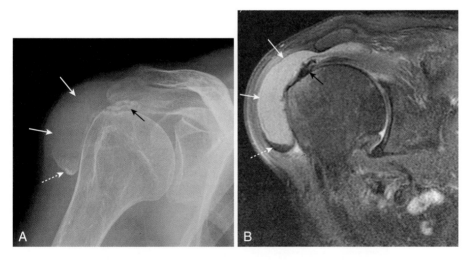

Fig. 3.5 (A) Anteroposterior (AP) radiograph of a patient with an acute inflammatory subdeltoid bursitis. There is soft tissue thickening *(white arrows)* due to bursal distention, with crystals collecting in the dependent portion of the bursa *(broken white arrow)*, originating from a focus of calcific tendinitis within the rotator cuff *(black arrow)*. (B) The corresponding coronal fat-saturated T2-weighted (FST2W) magnetic resonance image shows the same features with a high-signal intensity fluid-filled bursa *(white arrows)*, low-signal intensity crystals within the bursa *(broken white arrow)*, and the supraspinatus tendon *(black arrow)*. (From Waldman SD, Campbell RSD. *Imaging of Pain*. Philadelphia, PA: Saunders; 2011 [Fig. 99.2].)

patient's pain and aid in identification of fluid collection around the subdeltoid bursa as well as rice bodies (Figs. 3.6 and 3.7). Based on the patient's clinical presentation, additional testing may be indicated, including a complete blood count, erythrocyte sedimentation rate, and antinuclear antibody testing. Radionuclide bone scanning is indicated if metastatic disease or primary tumor involving the shoulder is a possibility. The injection technique described later serves as both a diagnostic and a therapeutic maneuver.

DIFFERENTIAL DIAGNOSIS

Subdeltoid bursitis is one of the most common causes of shoulder joint pain, and other painful conditions may mimic the clinical presentation of subdeltoid bursitis (Table 3.1). Osteoarthritis, rheumatoid arthritis, posttraumatic arthritis, and rotator cuff arthropathy are also common causes of shoulder pain that may coexist with subdeltoid bursitis. Less common causes of arthritis-induced shoulder pain include collagen vascular diseases, infection, villonodular synovitis, and Lyme disease. Acute infectious arthritis is usually accompanied by significant systemic symptoms, including fever and malaise, and should be easily recognized; it is treated with culture and antibiotics rather than with injection therapy. Collagen vascular diseases

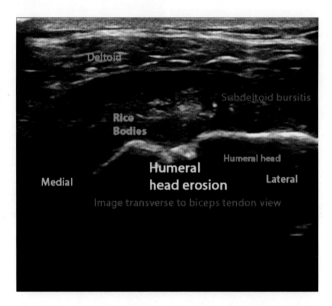

Fig. 3.6 Sonographic finding of subdeltoid bursitis in patient with mixed connective tissue disease. Note the rice bodies within the enlarged, fluid-filled subdeltoid bursa. (From Waldman SD. *Atlas of Common Pain Syndromes*. 4th ed. Philadelphia, PA: Elsevier; 2019 [Fig. 27.4].)

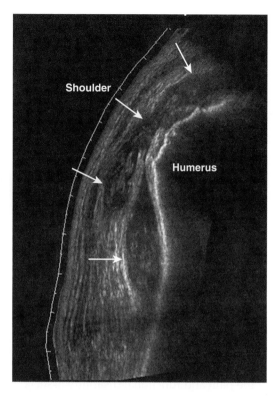

Fig. 3.7 Coronal panoramic ultrasound image of an infected subacromial bursa that is distended by low-echo fluid *(white arrows)* but contains areas of echogenic exudate. Rheumatoid arthritis might give a similar appearance, and infection was proved by aspiration. (From Waldman SD, Campbell RSD. *Imaging of Pain.* Philadelphia, PA: Saunders; 2011 [Fig. 99.3].)

TABLE 3.1 ■ Differential Diagnosis of Subdeltoid Bursitis

- Osteoarthritis
- Rheumatoid arthritis
- Posttraumatic arthritis
- Rotator cuff arthropathy
- Impingement syndromes
- Collagen vascular diseases
- Septic arthritis
- Villonodular synovitis
- Lyme disease

generally manifest as polyarthropathy rather than monoarthropathy limited to the shoulder joint; however, shoulder pain secondary to collagen vascular disease responds exceedingly well to the injection technique described here.

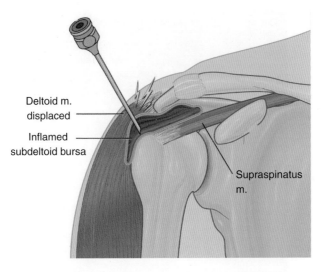

Deltoid m.
displaced

Inflamed
subdeltoid bursa

Supraspinatus
m.

Fig. 3.8   Proper needle placement for injection of the subdeltoid bursa. (From Waldman SD. *Atlas of Common Pain Syndromes*. 4th ed. Philadelphia, PA: Elsevier; 2019 [Fig. 27.6].)

TREATMENT

Initial treatment of the pain and functional disability associated with subdeltoid bursitis includes a combination of nonsteroidal antiinflammatory drugs (NSAIDs) or cyclooxygenase-2 inhibitors and physical therapy. Local application of heat and cold may also be beneficial. For patients who do not respond to these treatment modalities, injection of local anesthetic and steroid into the subdeltoid bursa is a reasonable next step.

Injection into the subdeltoid bursa is performed by placing the patient in the supine position and preparing the skin overlying the superior shoulder, acromion, and distal clavicle with antiseptic solution. A sterile syringe containing 4 mL of 0.25% preservative-free bupivacaine and 40 mg methylprednisolone is attached to a 1.5-inch, 25-gauge needle using strict aseptic technique. The lateral edge of the acromion is identified, and at the midpoint of the lateral edge, the injection site is identified. At this point, the needle is carefully advanced with a slightly cephalad trajectory through the skin and subcutaneous tissues beneath the acromion capsule and into the bursa (Fig. 3.8). If bone is encountered, the needle is withdrawn into the subcutaneous tissues and is redirected slightly more inferiorly. After the bursa is entered, the contents of the syringe are gently injected while the needle is slowly withdrawn. Resistance to injection should be minimal unless calcification of the bursal sac is present, in which case resistance to needle advancement is associated with a gritty feel. Significant calcific bursitis may ultimately require surgical excision to achieve complete relief of symptoms. After injection, the needle is removed, and a sterile pressure dressing and ice pack are applied to the injection site. Clinical case reports suggest that the injection of rilonacept, an interleukin-1 trap, may provide an alternative to the use of steroids in the treatment of subdeltoid bursitis. Ultrasound guidance may improve the accuracy of needle placement in patients in whom anatomic landmarks are hard to identify.

Physical modalities, including local heat and gentle range of motion exercises, should be introduced several days after the patient undergoes injection for shoulder pain. Vigorous exercises should be avoided because they will exacerbate the patient's symptoms.

HIGH-YIELD TAKEAWAYS

- The patient is afebrile, making an acute infectious etiology (e.g., septic arthritis) unlikely.
- The patient's symptomatology is the result of acute trauma, and physical examination and testing should be focused on the identification of ligamentous injury, acute arthritis, tendinitis, and bursitis.
- The patient has point tenderness over the deltoid muscle, which is highly suggestive of subdeltoid bursitis.
- There is warmth and swelling of the affected joint suggestive of an inflammatory process.
- The patient's symptoms are unilateral and only involve one joint, which is more suggestive of a local process than a systemic polyarthropathy.
- Sleep disturbance is common and must be addressed concurrently with the patient's pain symptomatology.
- Plain radiographs will provide high-yield information regarding the bony contents of the joint, but ultrasound imaging and MRI will be more useful in identifying soft tissue pathology.

Suggested Readings

Kang BS, Lee SH, Cho Y, et al. Acute calcific bursitis after ultrasound-guided percutaneous barbotage of rotator cuff calcific tendinopathy: a case report. *PM&R*. 2016;8:808–812.

Waldman SD. Subdeltoid bursitis and other disorders of the subdeltoid bursa. In: *Waldman's Comprehensive Atlas of Diagnostic Ultrasound of Painful Conditions*. Philadelphia, PA: Wolters Kluwer; 2016:206–213.

Waldman SD. Subdeltoid bursitis injection. In: *Atlas of Pain Management Injection Techniques*. 4th ed. Philadelphia, PA: Elsevier; 2017:147–150.

Waldman SD. The subdeltoid bursa. In: *Pain Review*. 2nd ed. Philadelphia, PA: Elsevier; 2017:91.

Wu T, Song HX, Dong Y, et al. Ultrasound-guided versus blind subacromial—subdeltoid bursa injection in adults with shoulder pain: a systematic review and meta-analysis. *Semin Arthritis Rheum*. 2015;45(3):374–378.

Taylor Severide

A 32-Year-Old Male With
Severe Right Shoulder Pain With
an Associated Catching
Sensation

- Learn the common causes of shoulder pain.
- Develop an understanding of the unique anatomy of the shoulder joint.
- Develop an understanding of the musculotendinous units that surround the shoulder joint.
- Develop an understanding of the bursae of the shoulder.
- Develop an understanding of the causes of bicipital tendinitis.
- Develop an understanding of the differential diagnosis of bicipital tendinitis.
- Learn the clinical presentation of bicipital tendinitis.
- Learn how to examine the shoulder.
- Learn how to use physical examination to identify bicipital tendinitis.
- Develop an understanding of the treatment options for bicipital tendinitis.

Taylor Severide

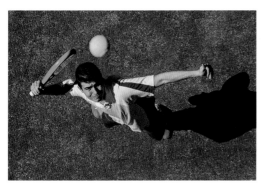

Taylor Severide is a 32-year-old male commercial real estate agent with the chief complaint of "I have a catch in my right shoulder and it hurts like hell." Taylor stated that he was competing in a paddleball tournament at his country club and thinks that this is what caused his shoulder problem. "Doc, the competition was really brutal, but I gave it my all. I was up against this guy in the semifinals and we were really evenly matched. The game went on for what seemed like hours and neither of us could bring the game home. It was match point and I served one as hard as I could and I felt something in the front of my right shoulder tear as I hit the ball. There was no way that guy was going to return that serve, but from then on the front of my shoulder has been hurting, especially in the mornings when I reach up to grab anything. I feel a catch and a sharp pain."

I asked Taylor about any antecedent shoulder trauma and he said no. I asked what made the pain better and he said that a couple of Aleves washed down with a couple of single malt whiskeys seemed to help. I asked Taylor what made it worse and he said the heating pad and washing and combing his hair. I asked how he was sleeping and he said, "Not worth a crap. I can't lay on my right side and that's the side I like to sleep on." He denied fever and chills. I asked Taylor to point with one finger where it hurt the most. He pointed to the anterior aspect of the right upper extremity just below the shoulder.

On physical examination, Taylor was afebrile. His respirations were 16, and his pulse was 72 and regular. He was normotensive with a blood pressure of 120/70. Taylor's head, eyes, ears, neck, throat (HEENT) exam was normal except for a tiny preauricular sinus on the right ear that looked like it had been infected and drained in the past (Fig. 4.1). His cardiopulmonary examination was normal. His thyroid was normal, as was his abdominal examination, which revealed no abnormal mass or organomegaly. There was no costovertebral angle (CVA) tenderness or peripheral edema. Taylor's low back examination was unremarkable. Visual inspection of the right shoulder was normal. I noted that Taylor was splinting his right shoulder by internally rotating his right upper extremity and holding it close to his side. The anterior right shoulder was a little warm but did not appear to be infected. There was marked point tenderness over the bicipital groove, and I thought I perceived a catching sensation when I asked Taylor to externally rotate his shoulder. Palpation of the bicipital groove was painful and

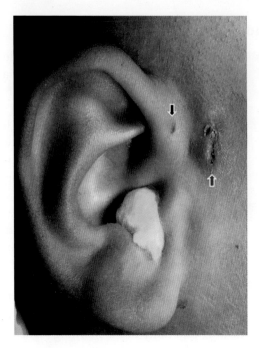

Fig. 4.1   Preauricular sinus *(black arrow)* with an abscess drainage slit *(red arrow)*. (From Wang L, Wei L, Lu L, et al. Excision of preauricular sinus with abscess drainage in children. *Am J Otolaryngol.* 2019;40(2):257–259.)

caused Taylor to wince in pain (Fig. 4.2). I performed a Yergason test and Speed test, which were both markedly positive on the right and negative on the left (Figs. 4.3 and 4.4). The left shoulder examination was normal, as was examination of his other major joints. A careful neurologic examination of the upper extremities revealed that there was no evidence of peripheral or entrapment neuropathy, and the deep tendon reflexes were normal.

Key Clinical Points—What's Important and What's Not

THE HISTORY

- A history of acute trauma following overhead serves while playing paddleball
- No history of previous significant shoulder pain
- No fever or chills
- Acute onset of shoulder pain following traumatic event with exacerbation of pain with shoulder use
- Pain in the right shoulder
- A catching sensation with elevation and external rotation of the right shoulder

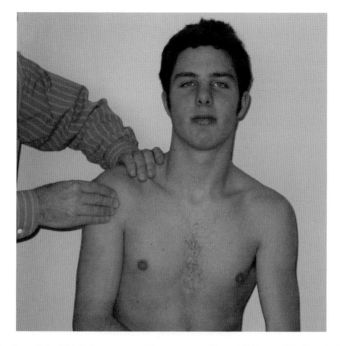

Fig. 4.2   Palpation of the bicipital groove and its contents. (From Waldman SD. *Physical Diagnosis of Pain: An Atlas of Signs and Symptoms*. 3rd ed. St Louis, MO: Elsevier; 2016 [Fig. 41.3].)

- Sleep disturbance
- Difficulty elevating and externally rotating the affected upper extremity

THE PHYSICAL EXAMINATION

- The patient is afebrile
- Point tenderness to palpation of the bicipital groove (see Fig. 4.2)
- Palpation of right shoulder reveals warmth to touch
- No evidence of infection
- Pain on range of motion, especially external rotation and elevation of the affected right shoulder
- The Yergason test was positive on the right (see Fig. 4.3)
- The Speed test was positive on the right (see Fig. 4.4)

OTHER FINDINGS OF NOTE

- Normal HEENT examination
- Preauricular sinus with suggestion of previous infection (see Fig. 4.1)
- Normal cardiovascular examination

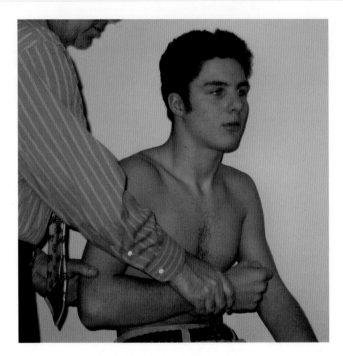

Fig. 4.3 The Yergason test for bicipital tendinitis. (From Waldman SD. *Physical Diagnosis of Pain: An Atlas of Signs and Symptoms*. 3rd ed. St Louis, MO: Elsevier; 2016 [Fig. 41.3].)

- Normal pulmonary examination
- Normal abdominal examination
- No peripheral edema
- Normal upper extremity neurologic examination, motor and sensory examination
- Examination of his other joints than the right shoulder were normal

What Tests Would You Like to Order?

The following tests were ordered:
- Plain radiographs of the right shoulder
- Ultrasound of the right shoulder, including the bicipital groove and its contents

TEST RESULTS

The plain radiographs of the right shoulder were negative. Ultrasound examination of the right shoulder revealed a significant effusion around the right bicipital tendon (Fig. 4.5).

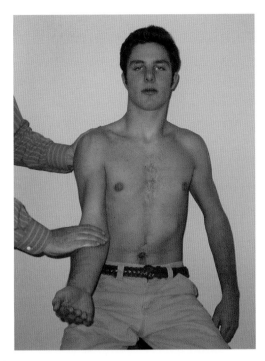

Fig. 4.4   The Speed test for bicipital tendinitis. (From Waldman SD. *Physical Diagnosis of Pain: An Atlas of Signs and Symptoms*. 3rd ed. St Louis, MO: Elsevier; 2016 [Fig. 42.1].)

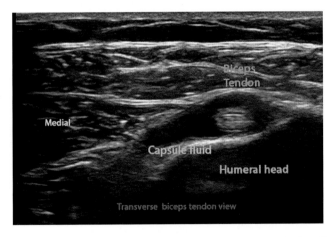

Fig. 4.5   Transverse ultrasound image demonstrating bicipital tendinitis with effusion. (Courtesy Steven Waldman, MD.)

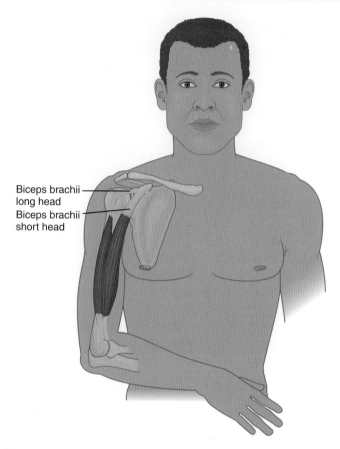

Biceps brachii
long head
Biceps brachii
short head

Fig. 4.6 The biceps tendon has a long and a short head, both of which are susceptible to the development of tendinitis. (From Waldman SD. *Atlas of Pain Management Injection Techniques*. 4th ed. St Louis, MO: Elsevier; 2017 [Fig. 35.4].)

 Clinical Correlation—Putting It All Together

What is the diagnosis?
- Bicipital tendinitis

The Science Behind the Diagnosis

ANATOMY

Along with the conjoined tendons of the rotator cuff, the bicipital muscle serves to stabilize the shoulder joint. The biceps muscle, which is named for its two heads, functions to supinate the forearm and flex the elbow joint (Fig. 4.6).

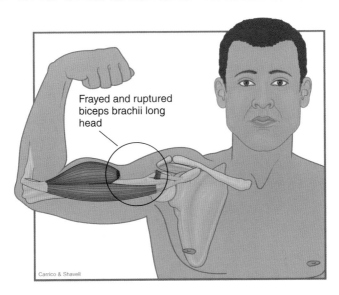

Frayed and ruptured
biceps brachii long
head

Carrico & Shavell

Fig. 4.7 Patients with rupture of the long head of the biceps muscle will demonstrate a positive Popeye deformity when the patient actively flexes the affected biceps muscle. (From Waldman SD. *Atlas of Pain Management Injection Techniques*. 4th ed. St Louis, MO: Elsevier; 2017 [Fig. 35.5].)

The long head finds its origin in the supraglenoid tubercle of the scapula, and the short head finds its origin from the tip of the coracoid process of the scapula. The long head exits the shoulder joint via the bicipital groove, where it is susceptible to trauma and the development of tendinitis. The long head fuses with the short head in the middle portion of the upper arm, forming the belly of the biceps muscle. The insertion of the biceps muscle is into the posterior portion of the radial tuberosity. The biceps muscle is innervated by the musculocutaneous nerve, which arises from the lateral cord of the brachial plexus. The fibers of the musculocutaneous nerve are derived from the C5, C6, and C7 nerve roots.

The biceps musculotendinous unit is subjected to significant stress during functioning, and misuse or overuse can result in inflammation and damage. If the damage remains untreated, the musculotendinous unit can rupture (Fig. 4.7). This most commonly occurs with the long head of the biceps, but the short head and the distal tendinous insertion can also rupture.

CLINICAL SYNDROME

The tendons of the long and short heads of the biceps are particularly susceptible to the development of tendinitis. Bicipital tendinitis is usually caused at least partially by impingement on the tendons of the biceps at the coracoacromial arch. The onset of bicipital tendinitis is generally acute, occurring after overuse or misuse of the shoulder joint, such as trying to start a recalcitrant lawn mower,

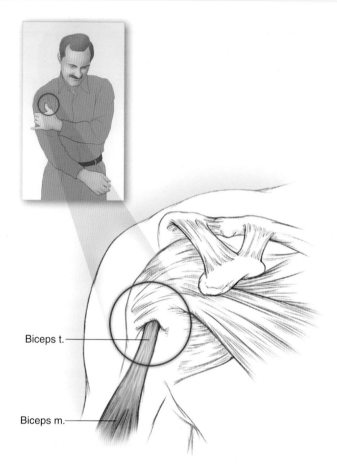

Biceps t.

Biceps m.

Fig. 4.8   Palpation of the bicipital groove exacerbates the pain of bicipital tendinitis. (From Waldman SD. *Atlas of Common Pain Syndromes*. 4th ed. Philadelphia, PA: Elsevier; 2019 [Fig. 28.1].)

practicing an overhead tennis serve, or performing an overaggressive follow-through when driving golf balls. The biceps muscle and tendons are susceptible to trauma and to wear and tear. If the damage is severe enough, the tendon of the long head of the biceps can rupture, leaving the patient with a telltale Popeye biceps (named after the cartoon character) (see Fig. 4.7). This deformity can be accentuated by having the patient perform the Ludington maneuver (i.e., placing both hands behind the head and flexing the biceps muscle).

SIGNS AND SYMPTOMS

The pain of bicipital tendinitis is constant and severe and is localized in the anterior shoulder over the bicipital groove (Fig. 4.8). A catching sensation may accompany the pain. Significant sleep disturbance is often reported. The patient

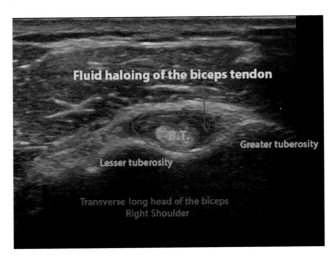

Fig. 4.9 Transverse ultrasound image of bicipital tendinitis. Note the positive halo sign indicating hypoechoic fluid surrounding the biceps tendon *(B.T.)*. (Courtesy Steven Waldman, MD.)

may attempt to splint the inflamed tendons by internal rotation of the humerus, which moves the biceps tendon from beneath the coracoacromial arch. Patients with bicipital tendinitis have a positive Yergason test—that is, production of pain on active supination of the forearm against resistance with the elbow flexed at a right angle (see Fig. 4.3). The Speed test may also be positive (see Fig. 4.4). Bursitis often accompanies bicipital tendinitis. In addition to pain, patients suffering from bicipital tendinitis often experience a gradual reduction in functional ability because of decreasing shoulder range of motion that makes simple, everyday tasks such as combing one's hair, fastening a brassiere, and reaching overhead quite difficult. With continued disuse, muscle wasting may occur, and a frozen shoulder may develop.

TESTING

Plain radiographs are indicated for all patients who present with shoulder pain. Based on the patient's clinical presentation, additional testing may be indicated, including a complete blood count, erythrocyte sedimentation rate, and antinuclear antibody testing. Magnetic resonance (MRI) and ultrasound imaging of the shoulder are indicated if rotator cuff tear is suspected and to further delineate the condition of the biceps tendons (Figs. 4.9 and 4.10; also see Fig. 4.5). Arthroscopy can aid in the diagnosis and treatment of bicipital tendinitis in selected patients, with the lipstick sign felt to be highly diagnostic for tendinitis of the long head of the biceps (Fig. 4.11). The injection technique described later serves as both a diagnostic and a therapeutic maneuver.

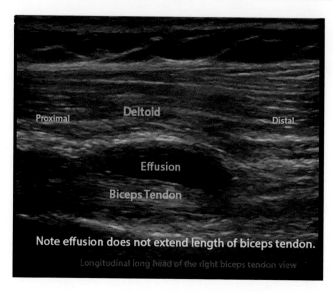

Fig. 4.10 Longitudinal ultrasound image demonstrating an effusion along a portion of the biceps tendon. (Courtesy Steven Waldman, MD.)

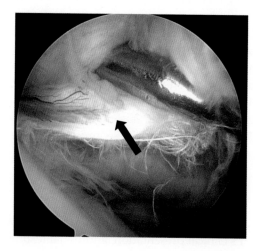

Fig. 4.11 The long head of the biceps tendon *(arrow)* should be retracted to evaluate the distal aspect for inflammatory and degenerative changes. Note the synovitis and fraying of the biceps tendon. The long head of the biceps tendon is inflamed and hyperemic within the bicipital groove, commonly referred to as the lipstick sign. (From Johnson JD, Edgar C. Suprapectoral biceps tenodesis. *Oper Tech Sport Med.* 2018;26(2):91−99.)

DIFFERENTIAL DIAGNOSIS

Bicipital tendinitis is usually a straightforward clinical diagnosis. However, coexisting bursitis or tendinitis of the shoulder from overuse or misuse may confuse the diagnosis. Occasionally, partial rotator cuff tear can be mistaken for bicipital tendinitis. In some clinical situations, consideration should be given to primary or secondary tumors involving the shoulder, superior sulcus of the lung, or proximal humerus. The pain of acute herpes zoster, which occurs before eruption of a vesicular rash, can also mimic bicipital tendinitis.

TREATMENT

Initial treatment of the pain and functional disability associated with bicipital tendinitis includes a combination of nonsteroidal antiinflammatory drugs (NSAIDs) or cyclooxygenase-2 (COX-2) inhibitors and physical therapy. Local application of heat and cold may also be beneficial. For patients who do not respond to these treatment modalities, injection with local anesthetic and steroid is a reasonable next step.

Injection for bicipital tendinitis is carried out by placing the patient in the supine position with the arm externally rotated approximately 45 degrees. The coracoid process is identified anteriorly. Just lateral to the coracoid process is the lesser tuberosity, which can be more easily palpated as the arm is passively rotated. The point overlying the tuberosity is marked with a sterile marker. The skin overlying the anterior shoulder is prepared with antiseptic solution. A sterile syringe containing 1 mL of 0.25% preservative-free bupivacaine and 40 mg methylprednisolone is attached to a 1.5-inch, 25-gauge needle using strict aseptic technique. The previously marked point is palpated, and the insertion of the biceps tendon is reidentified with the gloved finger. The needle is carefully advanced at this point through the skin, subcutaneous tissues, and underlying tendon until it impinges on bone. The needle is then withdrawn 1 to 2 mm out of the periosteum of the humerus, and the contents of the syringe are gently injected. The clinician should feel slight resistance to injection. If no resistance is encountered, either the needle tip is in the joint space itself or the tendon is ruptured. If resistance is significant, the needle tip is probably in the substance of a ligament or tendon and should be advanced or withdrawn slightly until the injection can proceed without significant resistance. The needle is then removed, and a sterile pressure dressing and ice pack are applied to the injection site. Recent clinical experience suggests that injection of platelet-rich plasma around the inflamed tendon may provide improved healing of tendinopathy. Ultrasound guidance may improve the accuracy of needle placement for patients in whom anatomic landmarks are hard to identify (Fig. 4.12).

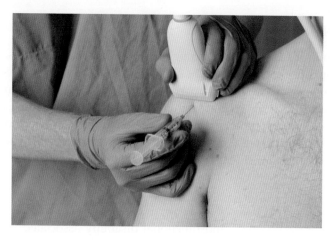

Fig. 4.12 Ultrasound-guided injection of the bicipital groove and its contents. (Courtesy Steven Waldman, MD.)

Physical modalities, including local heat and gentle range of motion exercises, should be introduced several days after the patient undergoes injection. Vigorous exercises should be avoided because they will exacerbate the patient's symptoms.

HIGH-YIELD TAKEAWAYS

- The patient is afebrile, making an acute infectious etiology (e.g., septic arthritis) unlikely.
- The patient's symptomatology is the result of acute trauma, and physical examination and testing should be focused on the identification of ligamentous injury, tendinitis, acute arthritis, and bursitis.
- The patient has point tenderness over the bicipital groove, which is highly suggestive of bicipital tendinitis.
- There is warmth over the affected joint, suggestive of an inflammatory process.
- The patient's symptoms are unilateral and only involve one joint, which is more suggestive of a local process than a systemic polyarthropathy.
- Sleep disturbance is common and must be addressed concurrently with the patient's pain symptomatology.
- Plain radiographs will provide high-yield information regarding the bony contents of the joint, but ultrasound imaging and MRI will be more useful in identifying soft tissue pathology.

Suggested Readings

Karistinos A, Paulos LE. Anatomy and function of the tendon of the long head of the biceps muscle. *Oper Tech Sports Med*. 2007;15(1):2—6.

McFarland EG, Borade A. Examination of the biceps tendon. *Clin Sports Med*. 2016;35(1):29—45.

Taylor SA, Fabricant PD, Bansal M, et al. The anatomy and histology of the bicipital tunnel of the shoulder. *J Shoulder Elbow Surg*. 2015;24(4):511—519.

Waldman SD. Bicipital tendinitis. In: *Atlas of Pain Management Injection Techniques*. 4th ed. Philadelphia, PA: Saunders; 2017:114—117.

Waldman SD. The biceps tendon. In: *Pain Review*. 2nd ed. Philadelphia, PA: Elsevier; 2017:91—92.

Waldman SD, Campbell RSD. Biceps tendinopathy. In: *Imaging of Pain*. Philadelphia, PA: Saunders; 2011:245—246.

Wu T, Song HX, Dong Y, et al. Ultrasound-guided versus blind subacromial—subdeltoid bursa injection in adults with shoulder pain: a systematic review and meta-analysis. *Semin Arthritis Rheum*. 2015;45(3):374—378.

Jules Landry

A 64-Year-Old Male With Severe Right Shoulder Pain With the Gradual Onset of Loss of Range of Motion

LEARNING OBJECTIVES

- Learn the common causes of shoulder pain.
- Develop an understanding of the unique anatomy of the shoulder joint.
- Develop an understanding of the musculotendinous units that surround the shoulder joint.
- Develop an understanding of the bursae of the shoulder.
- Develop an understanding of the causes of frozen shoulder.
- Develop an understanding of the differences between adhesive capsulitis and Milwaukee shoulder.
- Develop an understanding of the differential diagnosis of frozen shoulder.
- Learn to identify the underlying diseases associated with frozen shoulder.
- Learn the clinical presentation of frozen shoulder.
- Learn how to examine the shoulder.
- Learn how to use physical examination to identify frozen shoulder.
- Develop an understanding of the treatment options for frozen shoulder.

Jules Landry

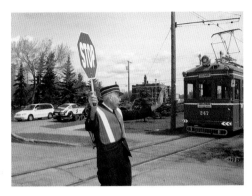

Jules Landry is a 64-year-old male crossing guard with the chief complaint of "I can't hold up my stop sign anymore." Jules stated that over the last several months, he has found it harder and harder to hold up his stop sign while working as a trolley crossing guard. He noted that the pain started as a dull, generalized ache of his right shoulder and that the pain was worse at night after a full day at work. He tried using a heating pad and extra-strength Tylenol without much success. Over time, Jules noted that the range of motion of his right shoulder continued to deteriorate, and the shoulder was painful all of the time. Currently, Jules noted, "Doctor, I can barely take care of myself. My wife has to shave me, and the only way I can hold up my stop sign is to brace my arm against my body. I'm afraid that a distracted driver won't see my stop sign and run into the trolley." I could see that Jules was really upset. I tried to reassure him that we would figure out what was going on and find a way to make it better.

Jules denied any antecedent trauma. I asked what made the pain better and he said, "Nothing really helps." I asked Jules what made his pain worse and he said, "Anything that requires me to use my arm—like my job!" I asked Jules how he was sleeping and he said, "I toss and turn all night long. My wife is making me sleep in the guest room because I keep waking her up." Jules denied fever and chills but reminded me that his "thyroid is low" and he "takes a thyroid pill every day." I asked Jules to point with one finger where it hurt the most and he responded, "There's no one place. The entire right shoulder hurts morning, noon, and night."

On physical examination, Jules was afebrile. His respirations were 18, and his pulse was 74 and regular. He was normotensive with a blood pressure of 126/74. Jules's (head, eyes, ears, neck, throat (HEENT) exam was normal, as was his cardiopulmonary examination. His thyroid was normal; specifically, no goiter was present and there were no classic findings of hypothyroidism (e.g., dry skin, hoarseness, facial puffiness) (Table 5.1). His abdominal examination revealed no abnormal mass or organomegaly. There was no costovertebral angle (CVA) tenderness or peripheral edema. Jules's low back examination was unremarkable. Visual inspection of the right shoulder was normal, although I noted that Jules was splinting his right upper extremity against his side to limit unintentional movement of the affected shoulder. There was no rubor or color of the right shoulder, but there was diffuse tenderness to deep palpation. Range of motion of

TABLE 5.1 ■ Signs and Symptoms of Hypothyroidism

- Fatigue
- Increased sensitivity to cold
- Dry skin
- Thinning hair
- Weight gain
- Puffy face
- Hoarseness
- Constipation
- Bradycardia
- Depression
- Goiter
- Muscle weakness
- Myxedema

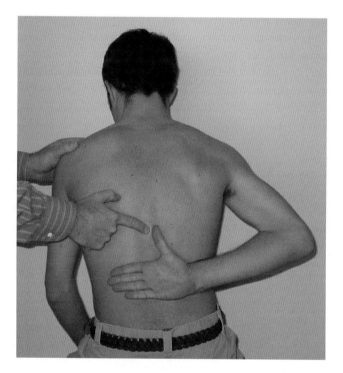

Fig. 5.1 The Apley scratch test for adhesive capsulitis. (From Waldman SD. *Physical Diagnosis of Pain: An Atlas of Signs and Symptoms*. 3rd ed. St Louis, MO: Elsevier; 2016 [Fig. 21.1].)

the right shoulder was extremely limited, and any attempt to move the shoulder met with strong objections from Jules. An Apley scratch test was positive on the right and negative on the left (Fig. 5.1). The left shoulder examination was normal, as was examination of his other major joints. A careful neurologic examination of the upper extremities revealed that there was no evidence of peripheral or entrapment neuropathy, and the deep tendon reflexes were normal.

Key Clinical Points—What's Important and What's Not

THE HISTORY

- A history of the gradual onset of right shoulder pain
- A history of a gradual decrease in the range of motion of the right shoulder
- A history of hypothyroidism
- An occupational history of holding an upper extremity in a specific position for long periods
- No history of previous significant shoulder pain
- No fever or chills
- Exacerbation of pain with shoulder use
- An increasing inability to carry out activities of daily living due to severe limitation of shoulder range of motion
- Sleep disturbance

THE PHYSICAL EXAMINATION

- The patient is afebrile
- There are no clinically obvious signs of hypothyroidism
- No evidence of infection
- Pain on range of motion of the right shoulder
- Extremely limited range of motion of the right shoulder
- The Apley scratch test was positive on the right (see Fig. 5.1)

OTHER FINDINGS OF NOTE

- Normal HEENT examination
- Normal cardiovascular examination
- Normal pulmonary examination
- Normal abdominal examination
- No peripheral edema
- Normal upper extremity neurologic examination, motor and sensory examination
- Examination of joints other than the right shoulder was normal

 What Tests Would You Like to Order?

The following tests were ordered:
- Plain radiographs of the right shoulder
- Arthrogram of the right shoulder
- Ultrasound of the right shoulder, including the bicipital groove and its contents
- Magnetic resonance imaging (MRI) of the right shoulder

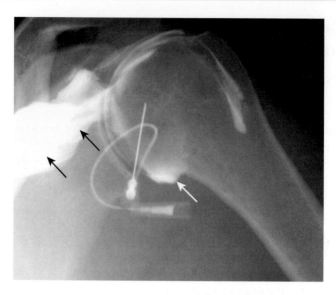

Fig. 5.2 Fluoroscopic image obtained during a distention arthrogram procedure in a patient with adhesive capsulitis. The axillary pouch is underdistended *(white arrow)* because of contraction of the joint capsule, and there is early extravasation of contrast medium from the joint *(black arrows)*. (From Waldman SD, Campbell RSD. *Imaging of Pain*. Philadelphia, PA: Saunders; 2011 [Fig. 94.1].)

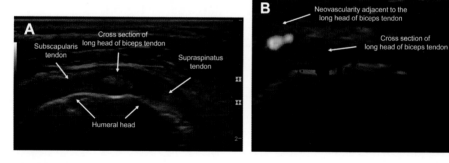

Fig. 5.3 Ultrasound of a patient with frozen shoulder. (A) Grayscale ultrasound scan of the rotator interval of the left shoulder. (B) Neovascularity adjacent to the long head of the biceps tendon. (From Lewis J. Frozen shoulder contracture syndrome—aetiology, diagnosis and management. *Man Ther.* 2015;20[1]:2—9.)

TEST RESULTS

The plain radiographs of the right shoulder were negative, but the arthrogram was markedly positive (Fig. 5.2). Ultrasound examination of the right shoulder revealed a significant thickening of the coracohumeral ligament and increased vascularity on Doppler ultrasound (Fig. 5.3). The MRI of the right shoulder

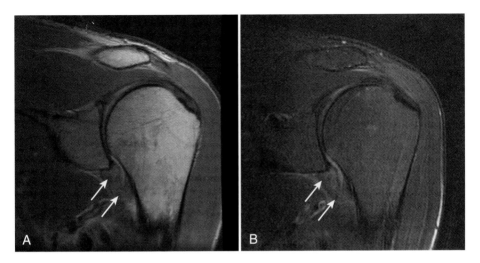

Fig. 5.4 Coronal proton density (A) and T2-weighted with fat suppression (FST2W) (B) magnetic resonance images in a different patient with adhesive capsulitis. There are thickening and high signal intensity within the inferior glenohumeral ligament and the capsule of the axillary pouch *(white arrows)*. Only a small joint effusion is present. (From Waldman SD, Campbell RSD, *Imaging of Pain*. Philadelphia, PA: Saunders; 2011 [Fig. 94.2].)

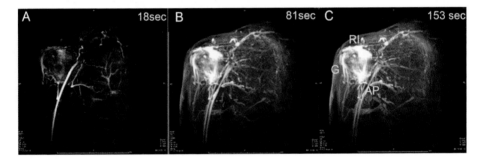

Fig. 5.5 Dynamic three-dimensional magnetic resonance imaging (3D MRI) findings of idiopathic severe frozen shoulder in the right shoulder of a 51-year-old woman. (A) At 18 seconds after the gadolinium intravenous injection (early phase). (B) At 81 seconds after the gadolinium intravenous injection (middle phase). (C) At 153 seconds after the gadolinium intravenous injection (late phase). There was abnormal enhancement at rotator interval *(RI)*, axillary pouch *(AP)*, and groove *(G)*. This abnormal enhancement is known as the burning sign. (From Sasanuma H, Sugimoto H, Fujita A, et al. Characteristics of dynamic magnetic resonance imaging of idiopathic severe frozen shoulder. *J Shoulder Elbow Surg.* 2017;26(2):e52–e57.)

revealed thickening of the inferior glenohumeral ligament and the capsule of the axillary pouch (Fig. 5.4). MRI three-dimensional dynamic testing with gadolinium administration revealed a positive burning sign consistent with frozen shoulder (Fig. 5.5).

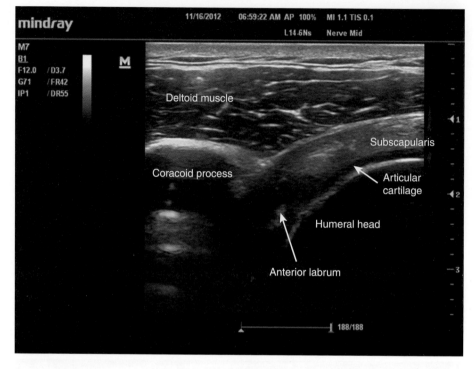

Fig. 5.6 Ultrasound anatomy of the glenohumeral joint. (From Waldman SD. *Physical Diagnosis of Pain: An Atlas of Signs and Symptoms*. 3rd ed. St Louis, MO: Elsevier; 2016 [Fig. 17.5].)

Clinical Correlation—Putting It All Together

What is the diagnosis?
- Frozen shoulder (adhesive capsulitis)

The Science Behind the Diagnosis

ANATOMY

The rounded head of the humerus articulates with the pear-shaped glenoid fossa of the scapula. The articular surface is covered with hyaline cartilage that is susceptible to arthritis. The rim of the glenoid fossa is composed of a fibrocartilaginous layer called the glenoid labrum, which is susceptible to trauma should the humerus be subluxed or dislocated (Fig. 5.6). The joint is surrounded by a relatively lax capsule that allows the wide range of motion of the shoulder joint at the expense of decreased joint stability. It is this capsule that, along with the shoulder ligaments, is most severely affected in frozen shoulder syndrome.

TABLE 5.2 ■ Adhesive Capsulitis Versus Milwaukee Shoulder

	Adhesive Capsulitis	Milwaukee Shoulder
Age	Fourth–sixth decade	Seventh decade
Gender	Female 60% Male 40%	Female 80% Male 20%
Laterality	Usually unilateral	Often bilateral
Knees Affected	No	Often
Rubor	No	Frequent
Color	No	Yes
Swelling/Effusion	No	Yes
Severe Pain	No	Yes
Antecedent Trauma	Sometimes	Frequent
Calcium Deposition Disease	No	Yes
Charcot Joint	No	Often
Hyperparathyroidism	No	Often
Dialysis Arthropathy	Rare	Often

The joint capsule is lined with a synovial membrane that attaches to the articular cartilage. This membrane gives rise to synovial tendon sheaths and bursae that are subject to inflammation. The shoulder joint is innervated by the axillary and suprascapular nerves.

The major ligaments of the shoulder joint are the glenohumeral ligaments in front of the capsule, the transverse humeral ligament between the humeral tuberosities, and the coracohumeral ligament, which stretches from the coracoid process to the greater tuberosity of the humerus. Along with the accessory ligaments of the shoulder, these major ligaments provide strength to the shoulder joint. The strength of the shoulder joint is also dependent on short muscles that surround the joint: the subscapularis, the supraspinatus, the infraspinatus, and the teres minor. These muscles and their attaching tendons are susceptible to trauma and to wear and tear from overuse and misuse.

CLINICAL SYNDROME

The term *frozen shoulder* describes a constellation of clinical symptoms, including the unilateral progressive limitation of passive and active range of motion of the shoulder and pain on range of motion. This term is used interchangeably with adhesive capsulitis by some clinicians, but in fact, adhesive capsulitis is just one class of frozen shoulder, with Milwaukee shoulder being the other (Table 5.2). The patient suffering from frozen shoulder will first note difficulty in reaching behind to fasten clothing such as a bra. Patients exhibit a positive Apley scratch test result; that is, they are unable to scratch their lower back with the affected extremity (see Fig. 5.1). The limitation of shoulder range of motion then progresses to limit the patient's ability to elevate the shoulder. The pain is constant, with worsening on use of the shoulder group. The pain is localized to the

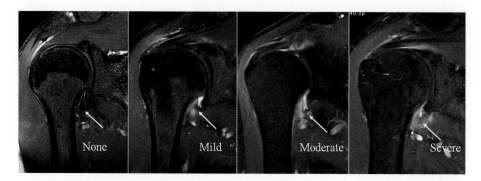

Fig. 5.7 The degree of enhancement of the axillary joint capsule *(arrows)* on contrast enhanced T1-weighted fat-suppressed oblique coronal images was classified as none, mild, moderate, and severe. (From Ahn K-S, Kang CH, Kim Y, et al. Diagnosis of adhesive capsulitis: comparison of contrast-enhanced MRI with noncontrast-enhanced MRI. *Clin Imag.* 2015;39(6):1061–1067.)

anterolateral aspect of the shoulder and may radiate into the lateral neck and upper anterior chest. Some patients report a grating or popping sensation with use of the joint, and crepitus may be present on physical examination. Frozen shoulder is distinguishable from other painful conditions of the shoulder such as tendinitis and bursitis in that the limitation of range of motion associated with frozen shoulder affects both passive and active range of motion, whereas tendinitis and bursitis affect only active range of motion.

Frozen shoulder is thought to be caused by a progressive adhesive capsulitis secondary to chronic inflammation of the structures of the shoulder (Fig. 5.7). Although coexistent tendinopathy or bursitis may be present, the inflammatory changes associated with frozen shoulder selectively affect the ligaments and joint capsule. Diseases that predispose the patient to the development of frozen shoulder can be divided into two general categories: (1) those that occur within the shoulder and proximal upper extremity (e.g., calcium deposition disease, rotator cuff tendinopathy, subdeltoid bursitis, biceps tendon tendinopathy, postimmunization shoulder pain), and (2) diseases that occur outside the shoulder region (e.g., stroke, diabetes, myocardial infarction, reflex sympathetic dystrophy, collagen vascular diseases). Regardless of the underlying cause of adhesive capsulitis, failure to quickly diagnose and treat this condition uniformly results in a poor clinical outcome.

Frozen Shoulder Secondary to Adhesive Capsulitis

Frozen shoulder secondary to adhesive capsulitis occurs more commonly in females in their fourth to sixth decades of life with the patient commonly complaining of pain that is localized around the shoulder and upper arm. Activity almost always makes the pain worse, with rest and heat providing some relief. The pain is constant and is characterized as aching in nature. Patients suffering from frozen shoulder will often complain of significant sleep disturbance as they are unable to lie on the affected shoulder. Some patients complain of a grating or popping sensation with use of the joint, and crepitus may be present on physical examination. The Apley scratch test will usually be positive with the patient unable to internally rotate the affected shoulder to scratch the midline of the back with an upward pointing thumb (see Fig. 5.1). Frozen shoulder secondary is usually unilateral, but can affect both shoulders at different times.

Frozen Shoulder Secondary to Calcium Crystal Deposition Disease— Milwaukee Shoulder

Patients suffering from frozen shoulder due to calcium crystal deposition disease will present clinically in a different manner than those patients whose etiology is adhesive capsulitis (see Table 5.2). Although both clinical syndromes occur more frequently in women, frozen shoulder secondary to crystal deposition disease, which is known as Milwaukee shoulder, has its average onset in the seventh decade of life. Unlike adhesive capsulitis, which is usually unilateral, Milwaukee shoulder is bilateral over 60% of the time, with the patients' knees often simultaneously affected. Although like frozen shoulder secondary to adhesive capsulitis, episodes of antecedent trauma or overuse can be identified, patients with Milwaukee shoulder frequently are suffering from calcium pyrophosphate deposition disease, hyperparathyroidism, Charcot arthropathy, and dialysis-associated arthropathy. Although some patients may experience a milder form of this disease, most patients experience a rapid progression of both pain and decreasing range of motion due to extensive destruction of the extraskeletal deposition of calcium crystals into the shoulder joint (Fig. 5.8). Radiographic, magnetic resonance, and ultrasound evaluations can reveal a striking amount of destruction of the articular cartilage and underlying bone of the glenohumoral joint, destruction of the coronoid, lysis of the distal clavicle, and calcification and tears of the musculotendinous units of the rotator cuff often resulting in a high riding humeral head (Fig. 5.9). Like the treatment of frozen shoulder secondary to adhesive capsulitis, treatment of Milwaukee shoulder is aimed at identifying and treating underlying diseases (e.g., hyperparathyroidism), the use of antiinflammatories (including short-course glucocorticoid therapy, intraarticular injections of local anesthetic and steroid—both as a diagnostic and therapeutic maneuver), manipulation under anesthesia, and extracorporeal shock wave therapy, all accompanied with aggressive physical and occupational therapy. Unfortunately, unlike the treatment of frozen shoulder secondary to adhesive capsulitis, which is usually successful, the treatment of Milwaukee shoulder is often disappointing despite everyone's best efforts.

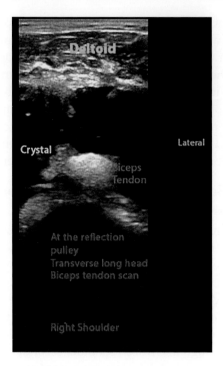

Fig. 5.8 Ultrasound image of right shoulder demonstrating crystal deposition in patient with Milwaukee shoulder. (Courtesy Steven Waldman, MD.)

SIGNS AND SYMPTOMS

In addition to pain, patients suffering from arthritis of the shoulder joint often experience a gradual reduction in functional ability because of decreasing shoulder range of motion, making simple everyday tasks such as combing one's hair, fastening a brassiere, or reaching overhead quite difficult. With continued disuse, muscle wasting may occur, and a frozen shoulder may develop. Sleep disturbance is quite common in patients suffering from adhesive capsulitis and may further exacerbate the patient's pain.

Patients suffering from frozen shoulder due to adhesive capsulitis will usually pass through four clinical stages that correlate with the progressive pathologic processes responsible for the patient's clinical symptomatology (Table 5.3). Stage 1, the aching stage, is characterized clinically as ill-defined shoulder pain that is localized to the deltoid region and associated with nighttime pain and some limitation of motion at the extremes of range. These symptoms are frequently misdiagnosed as osteroarthritis or mild tendinitis. Stage 1 is caused by hypertrophic synovitis, and arthroscopy will reveal a normal joint capsule and no obvious adhesions. At this stage of the disease, the pain and limited range of motion can

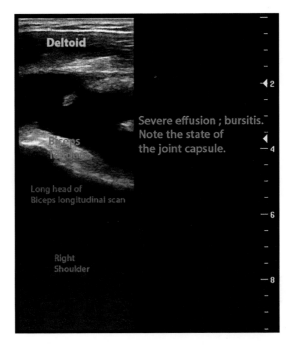

Fig. 5.9 Ultrasound image of the right shoulder demonstrating significant destruction of the gleno-humeral joint capsule with a massive joint effusion in patient with Milwaukee shoulder. (Courtesy Steven Waldman, MD.)

TABLE 5.3 ■ Stages of Adhesive Capsulitis

- Stage 1: Aching
- Stage 2: Freezing
- Stage 3: Frozen
- Stage 4: Thawing

be completely relieved by the administration of intraarticular local anesthetic. Stage 2, the freezing stage, presents clinically as severe shoulder pain, loss of external shoulder rotation, and stiffness that is caused by reactive synovitis and inflammatory changes of the periarticular tissues (Fig. 5.10). At this stage, limitation of range of motion can be improved but not fully corrected by the intraarticular administration of local anesthetic. Stage 3, the frozen stage, presents clinically as a marked reduction in shoulder range of motion and patient recognition of the significant reduction in the ability to carry out activities of daily living. The patient and clinician may misinterpret the decrease in pain intensity associated with improvement in spite of the severe functional limitations

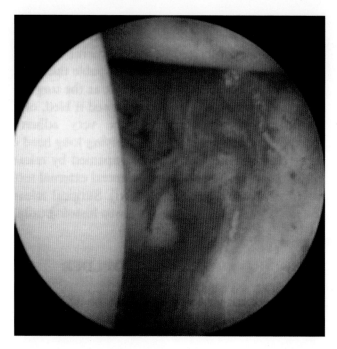

Fig. 5.10 Arthroscopy of the shoulder of a patient suffering from frozen shoulder demonstrating granulation tissue arising out of the subscapularis bursa at the origin of the biceps tendon, which is red, highly vascular, with a villous or fronded appearance of the synovium. (From Bunker T. Frozen shoulder. *Orthop Trauma*. 2011;25[1]:11–18.)

imposed by the disease. The frozen stage is due to significant pathologic thickening of the joint capsule (see Fig. 5.4). The intraarticular administration of local anesthetic will not improve the limitations of range of motion. Stage 4, the thawing stage, is characterized clinically by gradual return of shoulder function, although in many patients full recovery despite all treatment efforts remains elusive. Arthroscopy will reveal organized mature fibrotic adhesions within the joint space.

Clinically, the constellation of symptoms associated with Milwaukee shoulder looks very different from the presentation of Milwaukee shoulder. Milwaukee shoulder resembles the clinical presentation of acute gout (e.g., hot, swollen, extremely painful affected joints) and is hence called pseudogout. Large joint effusions are often present, and synovial fluid analysis will often reveal surprisingly low leukocyte counts, large numbers of erythrocytes, and basic calcium phosphate crystals, which are sometimes mixed with calcium pyrophosphate (known as apatite) (Fig. 5.11).

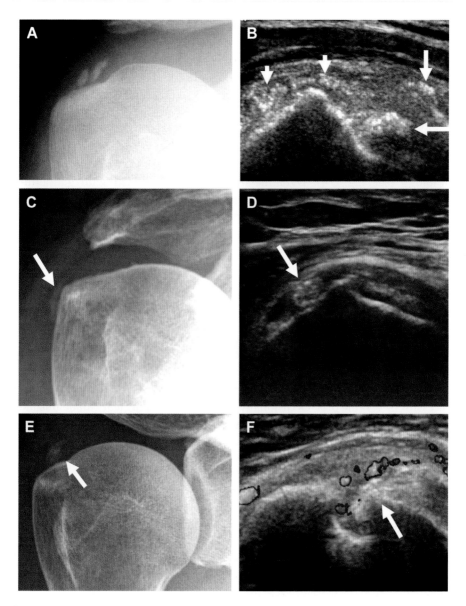

Fig. 5.11 Three cases of basic calcium phosphate (BCP) calcifications of the shoulder, with correlations between radiographs and ultrasound (US). (A, B) BCP calcification in resorptive phase. Radiograph (A) shows slightly blurry contours. US (B) shows multiple hyperechoic fragments visible *(arrows)*. Parts of the fragments are in the subacromial bursa *(short arrows)*. (C, D) BCP calcification that has migrated into the subacromial bursa *(arrows)*. Radiograph (C) shows faint calcification, whereas US (D) shows hyperechoic nodule. (E, F) BCP calcification that is migrating into the bone. Radiograph (E) shows calcification with blurry margins *(arrow* in E), especially on the inferior aspect. At US (F), a hyperechoic nodule is seen *(arrow* in F). The continuity of the calcification with bone erosion is clearly depicted. Hyperemic reaction at Doppler imaging is seen. Note that no shadowing is present in any of the cases of resorptive calcifications. (From Omoumi P, Zufferey P, Malghem J, et al. Imaging in gout and other crystal-related arthropathies. *Rheum Dis Clin N Am.* 2016;42[4]:621–644.)

TESTING

Plain radiographs are indicated for all patients who present with shoulder pain. Based on the patient's clinical presentation, additional testing may be indicated, including a complete blood count, erythrocyte sedimentation rate, thyroid testing, blood chemistries, and antinuclear antibody testing. Arthrography will provide significant information regarding the presence of adhesive capsulitis (see Fig. 5.3). Magnetic resonance and ultrasound imaging of the shoulder are indicated if frozen shoulder is suspected and to further identify other shoulder pathology (see Fig. 5.4). Dynamic three-dimensional MRI with gadolinium administration may be useful in further identifying a characteristic gadolinium "blush" known as the burning sign, which is thought to be diagnostic of frozen shoulder (see Fig. 5.5). Arthroscopy is extremely useful in the diagnosis and treatment of frozen shoulder (see Fig. 5.10). The injection technique described later serves as both a diagnostic and a therapeutic maneuver.

DIFFERENTIAL DIAGNOSIS

Frozen shoulder is usually a straightforward clinical diagnosis. However, coexisting bursitis or tendinitis of the shoulder from overuse or misuse may confuse the diagnosis. Adhesive capsulitis must be distinguished from Milwaukee shoulder, and a careful search for underlying diseases is important if treatment is to be successful (see Table 5.2). Occasionally, partial rotator cuff tear can be mistaken for bicipital tendinitis. In some clinical situations, consideration should be given to primary or secondary tumors involving the shoulder, superior sulcus of the lung, or proximal humerus.

TREATMENT

Initial treatment of the pain and functional disability associated with frozen shoulder includes a combination of nonsteroidal antiinflammatory drugs (NSAIDs) or cyclooxygenase-2 (COX-2) inhibitors and physical therapy. Local application of heat and cold may also be beneficial. For patients who do not quickly respond to these treatment modalities, injection with local anesthetic and steroid is a reasonable next step (Fig. 5.12). Physical modalities, including local heat and gentle range of motion exercises, should be introduced several days after the patient undergoes injection. Vigorous exercises should be avoided because they will exacerbate the patient's symptoms. For patients who continue to suffer decreased range of motion and pain, arthroscopy and manipulation of the shoulder under anesthesia to break up capsular adhesions should be considered sooner rather than later.

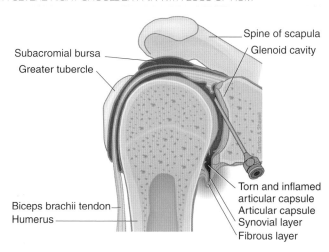

Spine of scapula
Glenoid cavity
Subacromial bursa
Greater tubercle
Torn and inflamed
articular capsule
Biceps brachii tendon
Articular capsule
Humerus
Synovial layer
Fibrous layer

Fig. 5.12 Proper needle position for injection of local anesthetic and steroid in the management of frozen shoulder. (From Waldman SD: *Atlas of Pain Management Injection Techniques*. 4th ed. St Louis, MO: Elsevier; 2017 [Fig. 45.2].)

HIGH-YIELD TAKEAWAYS

- The patient is afebrile, making an acute infectious etiology (e.g., septic arthritis) unlikely.
- The pain and limited range of motion is unilateral, making the diagnosis of frozen shoulder more likely than Milwaukee shoulder.
- The patient's symptomatology is significant, and physical examination and testing should be focused on the identification of underlying treatable conditions such as diabetes, hypothyroidism, and polymyalgia rheumatica.
- The patient has significant negative impact on his ability to carry out his activities of daily living and perform his job as a crossing guard.
- The patient's symptoms are unilateral and only involve one joint, which is more suggestive of a local process than a systemic polyarthropathy.
- Sleep disturbance is common and must be addressed concurrently with the patient's pain symptomatology.
- Plain radiographs will provide high-yield information regarding the bony contents of the affected joint, but arthrography, ultrasound imaging, and magnetic resonance imaging will be more useful in identifying soft tissue pathology and confirming the diagnosis of frozen shoulder.
- Intraarticular injection of local anesthetics and steroids should be carried out early in the course of the disease.

(Continued)

- Physical therapy should be initiated to preserve range of motion of the affected joint early in the course of the disease.

- Arthroscopy and manipulation of the affected joint under anesthesia should be considered in any patient who does not rapidly respond to intraarticular injection of steroid and local anesthetic and physical therapy.

Suggested Readings

Arkkila PE, Kantola IM, Viikari JS, et al. Shoulder capsulitis in type I and II diabetic patients: association with diabetic complications and related diseases. *Ann Rheum Dis*. 1996;55(12):907–914.

Cain EL, Kocaj SM, Wilk KE. Adhesive capsulitis of the shoulder. In: *The Athlete's Shoulder*. 2nd ed. Philadelphia, PA: Churchill Livingston; 2009:293–321.

Christian Reutter TR. Shoulder pain. In: *Decision Making in Pain Management*. 2nd ed. St Louis, MO: Mosby; 2006:160–162.

Dalton SE. Clinical examination of the painful shoulder. *Baillière's Clin Rheumatol*. 1989;3(3):453–474.

Davies AM. Imaging the painful shoulder. *Curr Orthop*. 1992;6(1):32–38.

Lee H-J, Lim K-B, Kim D-Y, et al. Randomized controlled trial for efficacy of intra-articular injection for adhesive capsulitis: ultrasonography-guided versus blind technique. *Arch Phys Med Rehabil*. 2009;90(12):1997–2002.

Raynor MB, Kuhn JE. Utility of features of the patient's history in the diagnosis of atraumatic shoulder pain: a systematic review. *J Shoulder Elbow Surg*. 2016;25 (4):688–694.

Waldman SD. Injection technique for frozen shoulder. In: *Atlas of Pain Management Injection Techniques*. 5th ed. Philadelphia, PA: Saunders; 2017:155–159.

Waldman SD, Campbell RSD. Adhesive capsulitis. In: *Imaging of Pain*. Philadelphia, PA: Saunders; 2011:239–240.

Jay Wilson

A 32-Year-Old Male With Acute Left Shoulder Pain

- Learn the common causes of shoulder pain.
- Develop an understanding of the unique anatomy of the shoulder joint.
- Understand the relationship of the muscles of the rotator cuff to the coracoacromial arch.
- Develop an understanding of the causes of supraspinatus tendinitis pain.
- Develop an understanding of the various types of rotator cuff injury.
- Learn the clinical presentation of supraspinatus tendinitis.
- Learn how to examine the shoulder.
- Learn how to use physical examination to identify pathology of supraspinatus tendinitis.
- Develop an understanding of the treatment options for supraspinatus tendinitis pain.

Jay Wilson

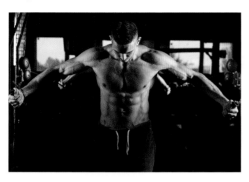

Jay Wilson is a 32-year-old male with the chief complaint of "my left shoulder is killing me." Jay stated that over the last 6 weeks, he began suffering from increasing pain in the left shoulder. He attributes the initial onset of pain to increasing his workout on the new cross-training machine at his gym. At first, he tried to work through it and when the pain kept getting worse, he began applying topical analgesic balm to his shoulder to no avail. I asked Jay if he had tried anything else to relieve his pain and he nodded and said, "Advil and an ice pack, but the Advil upset my stomach and the ice pack didn't help much."

I asked Jay if he had anything like this happen before. He shook his head and responded, "I have the usual aches and pains because I am always pushing myself to do more. I want to do the Ironman this summer and I have a long ways to go." I asked Jay what made his pain worse and he said, "Anytime I use my left shoulder, it really hurts, especially when reaching out or up to the side." Jay went on to say that sometimes when he used his left arm he would feel a sharp pain and catch in his shoulder. He said, "Doc, the crazy thing is that I feel like I am shrugging my left shoulder and I don't even realize that I'm doing it. It really looks kind of weird." Jay then complained that this pain was "really killing his workout" and messing with his sleep. "Every time I roll over to my left side, my shoulder wakes me up." I asked if he had any fever or chills and he shook his head no.

On physical examination, Jay was afebrile. His respirations were 16, and his pulse was 68 and regular. His blood pressure was 112/70. His head, eyes, ears, neck, throat (HEENT) exam was normal, as was his cardiopulmonary examination. His thyroid was normal. His abdominal examination revealed no abnormal mass or organomegaly. There was no costovertebral angle (CVA) tenderness. There was no peripheral edema. His low back examination was unremarkable. Visual inspection of the left shoulder revealed a small area of resolving ecchymosis anteriorly. I asked Jay to point with one finger where it hurts the most. He pointed to the area overlying the greater tuberosity of the left humerus. I noted that he was splinting the affected shoulder by elevating the left scapula, which gave him the shrugging appearance he mentioned. I asked Jay to abduct his right arm, which he did without difficulty. I asked him to repeat the maneuver on the left, and at about 90 degrees of abduction, he began to experience pain and further elevated his shoulder to compensate (Fig. 6.1). The left shoulder was a little warm but did not

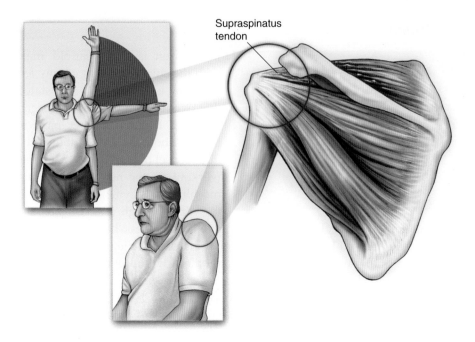

Supraspinatus
tendon

Fig. 6.1   Patients with supraspinatus tendinitis exhibit point tenderness of the greater tuberosity and a painful arc of abduction. (From Waldman SD. *Atlas of Uncommon Pain Syndromes*. 3rd ed. Philadelphia, PA: Saunders; 2014 [Fig. 28.1].)

appear to be infected. There was marked point tenderness over the left greater tuberosity. Jay exhibited a positive Dawbarn sign, which is pain to palpation over the greater tuberosity of the humerus when the arm is hanging down that disappears when the arm is fully abducted. Early in the course of the disease, passive range of motion is full and without pain (Fig. 6.2). The empty can test was also positive (Fig. 6.3). The right shoulder examination was normal, as was examination of his other major joints. A careful neurologic examination of the upper extremities revealed that there was no evidence of peripheral or entrapment neuropathy, and the deep tendon reflexes were normal.

Key Clinical Points—What's Important and What's Not

THE HISTORY

- A history of onset of severe left shoulder pain after heavy use of exercise equipment
- A history of worsening pain in spite of conservative therapy
- No history of previous significant shoulder pain

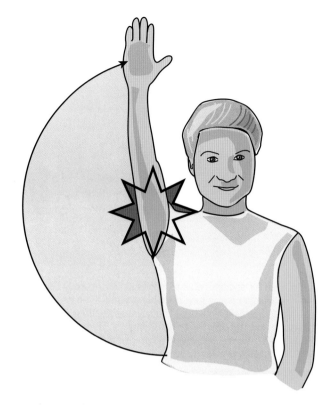

Fig. 6.2 Dawbarn sign is performed by having the patient hang the affected arm at the side while the examiner palpates the greater tuberosity of the humerus, which elicits pain. The patient's arm is then abducted while the examiner continues to palpate the greater tuberosity. The sign is considered positive and highly suggestive of supraspinatus tendinitis if the pain disappears when the arm is fully abducted. (From Waldman SD. *Physical Diagnosis of Pain: An Atlas of Signs and Symptoms*. 3rd ed. St Louis, MO: Elsevier; 2016 [Fig. 54.5].)

- No fever or chills
- Catching sensation in the right shoulder
- Sleep disturbance
- Difficulty abducting the affected left upper extremity

THE PHYSICAL EXAMINATION

- The patient is afebrile
- Palpation of right shoulder reveals point tenderness over the greater tuberosity of the humerus
- There is a painful arc of abduction
- Dawbarn sign is positive
- The empty can test is positive

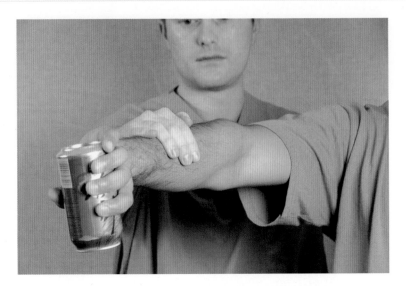

Fig. 6.3 The empty can test for supraspinatus tendonitis is performed by having the patient assume the standing position. The affected arm is then gradually elevated to 90 degrees in the scapular plane with the elbow fully extended and the arm in full internal rotation and the forearm pronated, as if the patient is trying to shake the last few drops out of an empty can. The examiner then exerts downward pressure to the affected arm. The test is considered positive if the patient experiences a significant increase in pain or demonstrates weakness. (Courtesy Steven Waldman, MD.)

- The shoulder is slightly warm to palpation
- No evidence of infection

OTHER FINDINGS OF NOTE

- Normal HEENT examination
- Normal cardiovascular examination
- Normal pulmonary examination
- Normal abdominal examination
- No peripheral edema
- Normal upper extremity neurologic examination, motor and sensory examination
- Examination of other joints was normal

 What Tests Would You Like to Order?

The following tests were ordered:
- Plain radiographs of the left shoulder, including anteroposterior (AP), lateral, and axillary views
- Ultrasound of the left shoulder

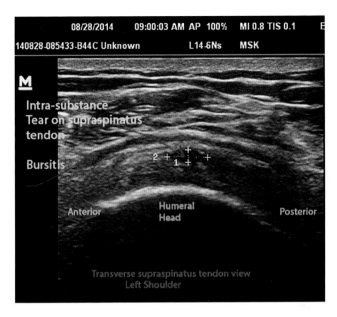

Fig. 6.4 Transverse ultrasound image demonstrating supraspinatus tendinopathy and bursitis as well as an intrasubstance tear of the supraspinatus tendon with the bursal contour preserved. (Courtesy Steven Waldman, MD.)

TEST RESULTS

The plain radiographs of the left shoulder revealed no evidence of bony abnormality. The ultrasound examination of the left shoulder revealed supraspinatus tendinitis and tendinopathy with an intersubstance tear of the supraspinatus tendon and associated bursitis (Fig. 6.4).

 ## Clinical Correlation—Putting It All Together

What is the diagnosis?
- Supraspinatus tendinitis

The Science Behind the Diagnosis

ANATOMY OF THE SUPRASPINATUS TENDON

The supraspinatus muscle serves to stabilize the shoulder by helping resist the inferior gravitational forces placed on the shoulder joint due to the downward pull from the weight of the upper limb. Responsible for the first 10 to 15 degrees of abduction of the upper extremity, the supraspinatus muscle abducts the arm at the shoulder by fixing the head of the humerus firmly against the glenoid fossa. The

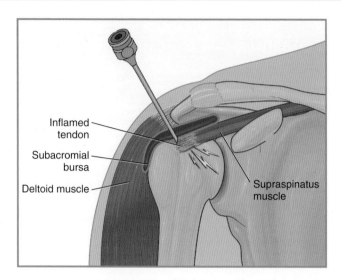

Fig. 6.5 The relationship of the supraspinatus muscle to the subacromial bursa and acromion. (From Waldman SD. *Atlas of Pain Management Injection Techniques*. 4th ed. St Louis, MO: Elsevier; 2017 [Fig. 28.3].)

supraspinatus muscle is innervated by the suprascapular nerve, which is comprised of fibers from the superior trunk of the brachial plexus. The muscle finds its origin from the supraspinous fossa of the scapula and inserts into the upper facet of the greater tuberosity of the humerus. The muscle passes across the superior aspect of the shoulder joint beneath the acromion, with the inferior portion of the tendon intimately involved with the joint capsule (Fig. 6.5). The musculotendinous unit is subject to impingement as it passes beneath the acromion (Fig. 6.6).

CLINICAL CONSIDERATIONS

Supraspinatus tendinitis can manifest as an acute or chronic painful condition of the shoulder. Acute supraspinatus tendinitis usually occurs in younger patients after overuse or misuse of the shoulder joint. Inciting factors may include carrying heavy loads in front of and away from the body, throwing injuries, or the vigorous use of exercise equipment. Chronic supraspinatus tendinitis tends to occur in older patients and to manifest in a more gradual or insidious manner, without a single specific event of antecedent trauma. The pain of supraspinatus tendinitis is constant and severe, with sleep disturbance often reported. The pain of supraspinatus tendinitis is felt primarily in the deltoid region. It is moderate to severe and may be associated with a gradual loss of range of motion of the affected shoulder. The patient often awakens at night when he or she turns over onto the affected shoulder.

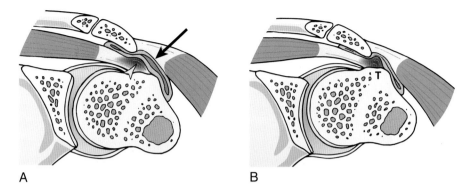

A   B

Fig. 6.6 (A) Drawing (coronal plane, cut section) of left shoulder during active elevation of arm halfway between flexion and abduction with hand in pronation explicitly depicts pooling of fluid in lateral aspect of subacromial-subdeltoid bursa *(arrow)* and alteration of normally convex surface of supraspinatus tendon *(arrowhead)* as arm is elevated. Supraspinatus tendon is not always involved in grade 2 subacromial impingement. There is also evidence of supraspinatus tendinosis and inflammatory changes in bursa. (B) Drawing (coronal plane, cut section) of left shoulder during active elevation of arm halfway between flexion and abduction with hand in pronation shows upward migration of humeral head in relation to glenoid cavity, which prevents passage of greater tuberosity *(T)* and soft tissue structures of supraspinatus outlet beneath acromion. (From El-Liethy N, Kamal H, Abdelwahab N, et al. Value of dynamic sonography in the management of shoulder pain in patients with rheumatoid arthritis. *Egyptian J Radiol Nuclear Med.* 2014;45(4):1171–1182 [Figs. 5, 6].)

SIGNS AND SYMPTOMS

A patient with supraspinatus tendinitis may attempt to splint the inflamed tendon by elevating the scapula to remove tension from the ligament, giving the patient a "shrugging" appearance (see Fig. 6.1). Point tenderness is usually present over the greater tuberosity. The patient exhibits a painful arc of abduction and complains of a catch or sudden onset of pain in the midrange of the arc, resulting from impingement of the humeral head onto the supraspinatus tendon. A patient with supraspinatus tendinitis exhibits a positive Dawbarn sign, which is pain to palpation over the greater tuberosity of the humerus when the arm is hanging down that disappears when the arm is fully abducted. Early in the course of the disease, passive range of motion is full and without pain (see Fig. 6.2). The empty can sign will also be positive (see Fig. 6.3).

TESTING

Plain radiographs are indicated in all patients who present with shoulder pain. Based on the patient's clinical presentation, additional testing, including

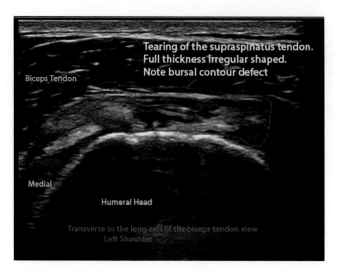

Fig. 6.7 Transverse ultrasound scan demonstrating full thickness, irregular tearing of the supraspinatus tendon with loss of the bursal contour. (Courtesy Steven Waldman, MD.)

complete blood cell count, sedimentation rate, and antinuclear antibody testing, may be indicated. Ultrasound and magnetic resonance imaging (MRI) of the shoulder is indicated if rotator cuff tear is suspected and to confirm the diagnosis of supraspinatus tendinitis (Figs. 6.7 and 6.8). The injection technique described here serves as a diagnostic and therapeutic maneuver.

DIFFERENTIAL DIAGNOSIS

Because supraspinatus tendinitis may occur after seemingly minor trauma or develop gradually over time, the diagnosis often is delayed. Tendinitis of the musculotendinous unit of the shoulder frequently coexists with bursitis of the associated bursae of the shoulder joint, creating additional pain and functional disability. This ongoing pain and functional disability can cause the patient to splint the shoulder group with resultant abnormal movement of the shoulder, which puts additional stress on the rotator cuff. This stress can lead to further trauma to the entire rotator cuff. With rotator cuff tears, passive range of motion is normal, but active range of motion is limited, in contrast to frozen shoulder, in which passive and active range of motion are limited. Rotator cuff tear rarely occurs before age 40 except in cases of severe acute trauma to the shoulder. Cervical radiculopathy rarely may cause pain limited to the shoulder, although in most instances, associated neck and upper extremity pain and numbness are present.

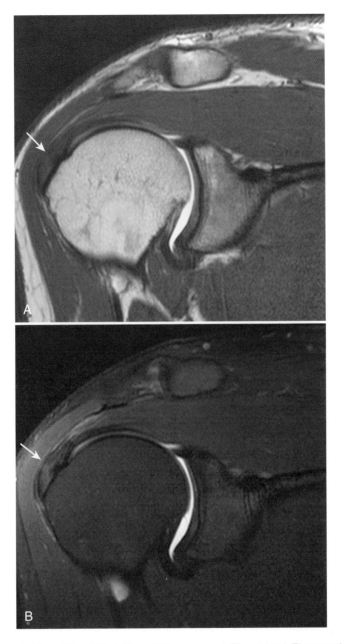

Fig. 6.8 Coronal oblique T1-weighted (A) and fat-suppressed T2-weighted (B) magnetic resonance images of a patient with supraspinatus tendinopathy. The distal tendon is thickened with increased signal intensity on both pulse sequences *(white arrows)*. There is no evidence of tendon tear. (From Waldman SD, Campbell RSD. *Imaging of Pain*. Philadelphia, PA: Saunders; 2011 [Fig. 91.2].)

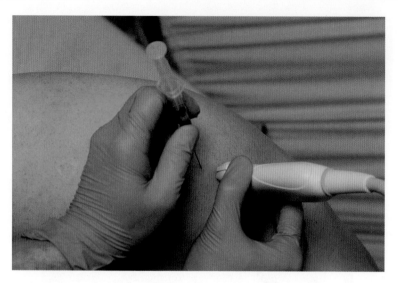

Fig. 6.9 Ultrasound-guided injection of the supraspinatus tendon. (Courtesy Steven Waldman, MD.)

TREATMENT

Initial treatment of the pain and functional disability associated with supraspinatus tendinitis should include a combination of nonsteroidal antiinflammatory drugs (NSAIDs) or cyclooxygenase-2 (COX-2) inhibitors and physical therapy. The local application of heat and cold also may be beneficial. For patients who do not respond to these treatment modalities, the following injection technique may be a reasonable next step. The use of physical therapy, including gentle range of motion exercises, should be introduced several days after the patient undergoes this injection technique for shoulder pain. Vigorous exercises should be avoided because they would exacerbate the symptoms. To inject the supraspinatus tendon, the patient is placed in the supine position, with the forearm medially rotated behind the back. This positioning of the upper extremity places the lateral epicondyle of the elbow in an anterior position and makes its identification easier. After identification of the lateral epicondyle of the elbow, the humerus is traced superiorly to the anterior edge of the acromion. A slight indentation just below the anterior edge of the acromion marks the point of insertion of the supraspinatus tendon into the upper facet of the greater tuberosity of the humerus (Fig. 6.9; see also Fig. 6.5).

HIGH-YIELD TAKEAWAYS

- The patient is afebrile, making an acute infectious etiology (e.g., septic arthritis) unlikely.
- The patient's symptomatology is the result of acute trauma, and physical examination and testing should be focused on the identification of ligamentous injury and fracture.
- The patient's pain is localized to the acromioclavicular joint.
- The patient's symptoms are unilateral and only involve one joint, which is more suggestive of a local process than a systemic polyarthropathy.
- Sleep disturbance is common and must be addressed concurrently with the patient's pain symptomatology.
- Plain radiographs will provide high-yield information regarding the bony contents of the joint, but ultrasound imaging and MRI will be more useful in identifying soft tissue pathology.

Suggested Readings

Allen H, Chan BY, Davis KW, et al. Overuse injuries of the shoulder. *Radiol Clin N Am.* 2019;57(5):897−909.

Cibulas A, Leyva A, Cibulas G, et al. Acute shoulder injury. *Radiol Clin N Am.* 2019;57(5):883−896.

Netter FH. Shoulder (glenohumeral joint). In: *Atlas of Human Anatomy.* 4th ed. Philadelphia, PA: Saunders; 2006.

Reschke D, Dagrosa R, Matteson DT. An unusual cause of shoulder pain and weakness. *Am J Emerg Med.* 2018;36(12):2339.e5−2339.e6.

Waldman SD. *Atlas of Pain Management Injection Techniques.* 4th ed. Philadelphia, PA: Saunders; 2017:94−97.

Waldman SD. Clinical correlates: functional anatomy of the shoulder. In: *Physical Diagnosis of Pain: An Atlas of Signs and Symptoms.* 3rd ed. Philadelphia, PA: Saunders; 2016.

Waldman SD. Rotator cuff tear. In: Waldman SD, ed. *Atlas of Common Pain Syndromes.* 4th ed. Philadelphia, PA: Elsevier; 2019:129−133.

Patrick Holmes

A 27-Year-Old Male With Acute Right Shoulder and Scapular Pain

- Learn the common causes of shoulder pain.
- Develop an understanding of the unique anatomy of the shoulder joint.
- Understand the function of the muscles of the rotator cuff.
- Develop an understanding of the causes of infraspinatus tendinitis pain.
- Develop an understanding of the various types of rotator cuff injury.
- Learn the clinical presentation of infraspinatus tendinitis.
- Learn how to examine the shoulder.
- Learn how to use physical examination to identify pathology of infraspinatus tendinitis.
- Develop an understanding of the treatment options for infraspinatus tendinitis pain.

Patrick Holmes

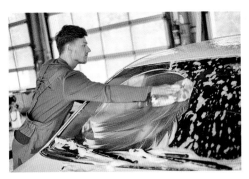

Patrick Holmes is a 27-year-old male car detailer with the chief complaint of "I have pain and a catch in the back of my right shoulder." Patrick stated that over the last 3 weeks, he worked several double shifts in a row to fill in for a sick coworker. He went on to state that it was the first patch of good weather after a couple of weeks of ice and snow, so the car wash was especially busy. He began to notice pain that was located in the back of the right shoulder when he would reach up to clean windshields, especially on the big SUVs. He tried a heating pad and Tylenol, but the pain continued to get worse. I asked Patrick if he had ever had anything like this before and he shook his head no. I asked what made it better and he said he had been "pulling his right shoulder back to take the pressure off." Patrick noted that it was getting harder and harder to raise his arm out to the side to do his job, which was really worrying him because "a man has to work if he wants to eat." I asked how he was sleeping and he said that he had taken to sleeping in his recliner because every time he rolled over onto his right shoulder in bed, it woke him up. Patrick denied any fever or chills.

On physical examination, Patrick was afebrile. His respirations were 16, and his pulse was 68 and regular. His blood pressure was 118/72. His head, eyes, ears, neck, throat (HEENT) exam was normal, as was his cardiopulmonary examination. His thyroid was normal. His abdominal examination revealed no abnormal mass or organomegaly. There was no costovertebral angle (CVA) tenderness. There was no peripheral edema. His low back examination was unremarkable. Visual inspection of the right shoulder was unremarkable. I asked Patrick to point with one finger where it hurt the most, and he pointed to the area overlying the point at which the infraspinatus musculotendinous unit attaches to the middle facet of the greater tuberosity of the right humerus. I noted that he was in fact splinting the affected shoulder by pulling the right scapula posteriorly (Fig. 7.1). I asked Patrick to abduct his left arm, which he did without any difficulty. I asked him to repeat the maneuver on the right, and at about 90 degrees of abduction, he began to experience pain and was very resistant to abducting the arm any further (Fig. 7.2). The right shoulder was a little warm but did not appear to be infected. There was marked point tenderness at the point where the infraspinatus musculotendinous unit attached to the middle facet of the greater tuberosity of the right humerus. Patrick exhibited a positive midarc abduction test, which is performed by having the patient abduct the arm until the point at which the pain begins.

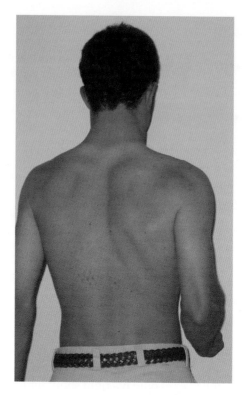

Fig. 7.1 The patient with infraspinatus tendinitis will unconsciously pull the affected shoulder back-wards to take the pressure off the insertion of the infraspinatus muscle. (From Waldman SD. *Physical Diagnosis of Pain: An Atlas of Signs and Symptoms*. 3rd ed. St Louis, MO: Elsevier; 2016 [Fig. 57.2].)

The patient is then asked to continue abducting the arm. The test is positive if the patient lowers the contralateral shoulder to further elevate the affected arm with-out further abduction (Fig. 7.3). Patrick's left shoulder examination was normal, as was examination of his other major joints. A careful neurologic examination of the upper extremities revealed that there was no evidence of peripheral or entrap-ment neuropathy, and the deep tendon reflexes were normal.

Key Clinical Points—What's Important and What's Not

THE HISTORY

- A history of onset of severe right shoulder pain after overuse of the right shoulder while working as a car detailer at a car wash
- A history of worsening pain in spite of conservative therapy
- No history of previous significant shoulder pain
- No fever or chills

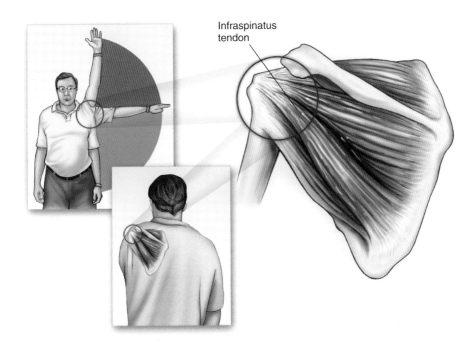

Fig. 7.2 Patients with infraspinatus tendinitis exhibit posterior point tenderness and a painful arc of abduction. (From Waldman SD. *Atlas of Uncommon Pain Syndromes*. 3rd ed. Philadelphia, PA: Saunders; 2014 [Fig. 29.1].)

- Catching sensation and pain in the right shoulder with abduction and posterior movement
- Sleep disturbance
- Difficulty abducting the affected right upper extremity

THE PHYSICAL EXAMINATION

- The patient is afebrile
- Palpation of right shoulder reveals point tenderness posteriorly over the point of insertion of the infraspinatus muscle on the middle facet of the greater tuberosity of the humerus
- There is a painful arc of abduction
- Midarc abduction sign is positive

OTHER FINDINGS OF NOTE

- Normal HEENT examination
- Normal cardiovascular examination
- Normal pulmonary examination

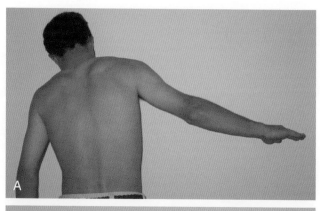

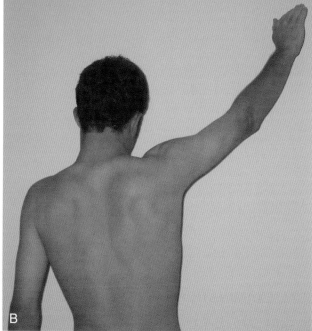

Fig. 7.3 (A) The midarc abduction test for infraspinatus tendinitis is performed by having the patient abduct the arm until the point at which the pain begins. (B) The patient is then asked to continue abducting the arm. The test is positive if the patient lowers the contralateral shoulder to further elevate the affected arm without further abduction. (From Waldman SD. *Physical Diagnosis of Pain: An Atlas of Signs and Symptoms*. 3rd ed. St Louis, MO: Elsevier; 2016 [Fig. 57.3].)

- Normal abdominal examination
- No peripheral edema
- Normal upper extremity neurologic examination, motor and sensory examination
- Examination of other joints was normal

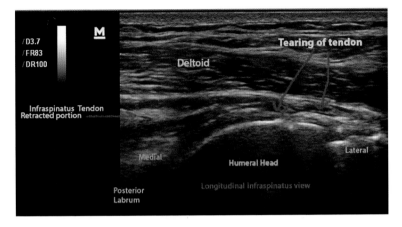

Fig. 7.4 Longitudinal ultrasound view of tearing of the infraspinatus tendon. Note the retracted portion of the tendon. (Courtesy Steven Waldman, MD.)

 What Tests Would You Like to Order?

The following tests were ordered:
- Plain radiographs of the right shoulder, including anteroposterior (AP), lateral, axillary views
- Ultrasound of the right shoulder

TEST RESULTS

The plain radiographs of the right shoulder revealed no evidence of bony abnormality. The ultrasound examination of the right shoulder revealed tearing of the infraspinatus tendon with retraction of the proximal tendon (Fig. 7.4).

 Clinical Correlation—Putting It All Together

What is the diagnosis?
- Infraspinatus tendinitis

The Science Behind the Diagnosis
ANATOMY OF THE INFRASPINATUS TENDON

The infraspinatus muscle, as part of the rotator cuff, provides shoulder stability (Fig. 7.5). In conjunction with the teres minor muscle, the infraspinatus muscle

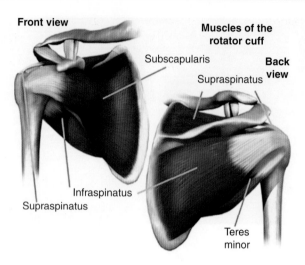

Fig. 7.5 The musculotendinous units of the rotator cuff. (From Vollans S, Ali A. Rotator cuff tears. *Surgery (Oxford)*. 2016;34(3):129–133.)

externally rotates the arm at the shoulder. Like the supraspinatus muscle, the infraspinatus muscle is innervated by the suprascapular nerve, which is comprised of fibers from the superior trunk of the brachial plexus. The infraspinatus muscle finds its origin in the infraspinous fossa of the scapula and inserts into the middle facet of the greater tuberosity of the humerus (see Fig. 7.2). It is at this insertion on the greater tuberosity that infraspinatus tendinitis and tendinopathy most commonly occur.

CLINICAL CONSIDERATIONS

Infraspinatus tendinitis can manifest as an acute or chronic painful condition of the shoulder. Acute infraspinatus tendinitis usually occurs in a younger group of patients after overuse or misuse of the shoulder joint. Inciting factors include activities that require repeated abduction and lateral rotation of the humerus, such as installing brake pads during assembly-line work. The vigorous use of exercise equipment also has been implicated. The pain of infraspinatus tendinitis is constant, severe, and localized to the deltoid area. Significant sleep disturbance is often reported. Patients with infraspinatus tendinitis exhibit pain with lateral rotation of the humerus and on active abduction. Chronic infraspinatus tendinitis tends to occur in older patients and to manifest in a more gradual or insidious manner, without a single specific event of antecedent trauma. The pain of infraspinatus tendinitis may be associated with a gradual loss of range of motion of the affected shoulder. The patient often awakens at night when rolling over onto the affected shoulder.

SIGNS AND SYMPTOMS

The patient may attempt to splint the inflamed infraspinatus tendon by rotating the scapula posteriorly to remove tension from the tendon (see Fig. 7.2). Point tenderness is usually present over the greater tuberosity. The patient exhibits a painful arc of abduction and complains of a catch or sudden onset of pain in the midrange of the arc. Early in the course of the disease, passive range of motion is full and painless. As the disease progresses, patients with infraspinatus tendinitis often experience a gradual decrease in functional ability with decreasing shoulder range of motion, making simple everyday tasks such as combing hair, fastening a brassiere, or reaching overhead quite difficult. With continued disuse, muscle wasting may occur and a frozen shoulder may develop.

TESTING

Plain radiographs are indicated in all patients with shoulder pain. Based on the patient's clinical presentation, additional testing, including complete blood cell count, erythrocyte sedimentation rate, and antinuclear antibody testing, may be indicated. Ultrasound and magnetic resonance imaging (MRI) of the shoulder is indicated if rotator cuff tear is suspected as well as to confirm the diagnosis of infraspinatus tendinitis and to identify other shoulder pathology (Fig. 7.6). The injection technique discussed here serves as a diagnostic and therapeutic maneuver.

DIFFERENTIAL DIAGNOSIS

Because infraspinatus tendinitis may occur after seemingly minor trauma or develop gradually over time, the diagnosis is often delayed. Tendinitis of the musculotendinous unit of the shoulder frequently coexists with bursitis of the associated bursae of the shoulder joint, creating additional pain and functional disability. This ongoing pain and functional disability can cause the patient to splint the shoulder group, with resultant abnormal movement of the shoulder that puts additional stress on the rotator cuff. This stress can lead to further trauma to the entire rotator cuff. With rotator cuff tears, passive range of motion is normal, but active range of motion is limited, in contrast to frozen shoulder, in which passive and active range of motion are limited. Rotator cuff tear rarely

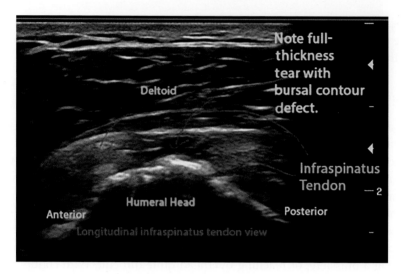

Fig. 7.6   Ultrasound image demonstrating full-thickness tear of the infraspinatus tendon. Note the bursal contour defect. (Courtesy Steven Waldman, MD.)

occurs before age 40 except in cases of severe acute trauma to the shoulder. Cervical radiculopathy rarely may cause pain limited to the shoulder, although in most instances associated neck and upper extremity pain and numbness are present.

TREATMENT

Initial treatment of the pain and functional disability associated with rotator cuff tear should include a combination of nonsteroidal antiinflammatory drugs (NSAIDs) or cyclooxygenase-2 (COX-2) inhibitors and physical therapy. The local application of heat and cold also may be beneficial. For patients who do not respond to these treatment modalities, the following injection technique may be a reasonable next step. The use of physical therapy, including gentle range of motion exercises, should be introduced several days after the patient undergoes this injection technique for shoulder pain. Vigorous exercises should be avoided because they would exacerbate the symptoms.

To inject the infraspinatus tendon, the skin overlying the posterior shoulder is prepared with antiseptic solution. A sterile syringe containing 1 mL of 0.25% preservative-free bupivacaine and 40 mg of methylprednisolone is attached to a 25-gauge, 1.5-inch needle, using strict aseptic technique. With strict aseptic technique, the previously marked point is palpated, and the insertion of the infraspinatus tendon is identified again with the gloved finger. The needle is carefully advanced at this point through the skin and subcutaneous tissues, and the

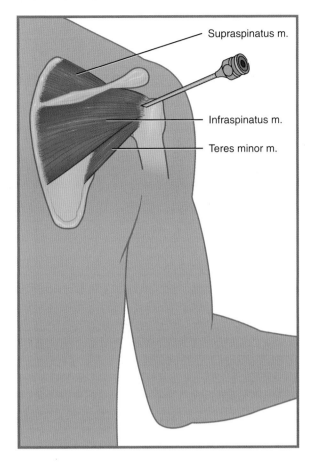

Fig. 7.7   Correct needle placement for injection into the infraspinatus tendon. (From Waldman SD: *Atlas of Pain Management Injection Techniques*. 4th ed. St Louis, MO: Elsevier; 2017 [Fig. 29.3].)

margin of the deltoid muscle and underlying infraspinatus muscle until it impinges on bone (Fig. 7.7). The needle is withdrawn 1 to 2 mm out of the periosteum of the humerus, and the contents of the syringe are gently injected. There should be slight resistance to injection. If no resistance is encountered, either the needle tip is in the joint space itself or the infraspinatus tendon is ruptured. If significant resistance to injection is felt, the needle tip is probably in the substance of a ligament or tendon and should be advanced or withdrawn slightly until the injection proceeds without significant resistance. The needle is removed, and a sterile pressure dressing and ice pack are placed at the injection site. Ultrasound-guided injection may improve the accuracy of needle placement in selected patients (Fig. 7.8).

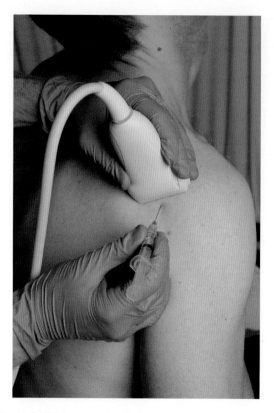

Fig. 7.8 Ultrasound-guided injection may improve the accuracy of needle placement in selected patients. (Courtesy Steven Waldman, MD.)

HIGH-YIELD TAKEAWAYS

- The patient is afebrile, making an acute infectious etiology (e.g., septic arthritis) unlikely.
- The patient's symptomatology is the result of acute overuse of the musculotendinous units of the shoulder, and physical examination and testing should be focused on the identification of ligamentous injury and fracture.
- The patient's pain is localized to the insertion of the infraspinatus tendon.
- The patient's symptoms are unilateral and only involve one joint, which is more suggestive of a local process than a systemic polyarthropathy.
- Sleep disturbance is common and must be addressed concurrently with the patient's pain symptomatology.
- Plain radiographs will provide high-yield information regarding the bony contents of the joint, but ultrasound imaging and MRI will be more useful in identifying soft tissue pathology.

Suggested Readings

Allen H, Chan BY, Davis KW, et al. Overuse injuries of the shoulder. *Radiol Clin N Am.* 2019;57(5):897−909.

Cibulas A, Leyva A, Cibulas G, et al. Acute shoulder injury. *Radiol Clin N Am.* 2019;57(5):883−897.

Netter FH. Shoulder (glenohumeral joint). In: *Atlas of Human Anatomy.* 4th ed. Philadelphia, PA: Saunders; 2007.

Reschke D, Dagrosa R, Matteson DT. An unusual cause of shoulder pain and weakness. *Am J Emerg Med.* 2018;37(12):2339.e5−2339.e7.

Waldman SD. *Atlas of Pain Management Injection Techniques.* 4th ed. Philadelphia, PA: Saunders; 2017:94−97.

Waldman SD. Clinical correlates: functional anatomy of the shoulder. In: *Physical Diagnosis of Pain: An Atlas of Signs and Symptoms.* 3rd ed. Philadelphia, PA: Saunders; 2017.

Waldman SD. Rotator cuff tear. In: *Atlas of Common Pain Syndromes.* 4th ed. Philadelphia, PA: Elsevier; 2019:129−133.

David "Tommy" John

A 32-Year-Old Male With Acute Right Shoulder Pain and an Inability to Raise His Right Upper Extremity

- Learn the common causes of shoulder pain.
- Develop an understanding of the unique anatomy of the shoulder joint.
- Develop an understanding of the anatomy of the rotator cuff.
- Understand the function of the muscles of the rotator cuff.
- Develop an understanding of the causes of rotator cuff tear.
- Develop an understanding of the various types of rotator cuff injury.
- Learn the clinical presentation of rotator cuff tear.
- Learn how to examine the shoulder.
- Learn how to use physical examination to identify pathology of the rotator cuff.
- Develop an understanding of the treatment options for rotator cuff tear.

David "Tommy" John

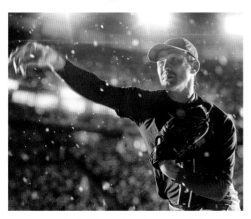

"My name is David, but my friends call me 'Tommy,'" said my new patient as I introduced myself to him. When I gave him a blank look he said, "You know, Doc, Tommy John, after the great pitcher." I said, "Oh, yeah, but I thought that Tommy John was the name of some type of arm surgery, but who knew?" David "Tommy" John was a 32-year-old baseball pitcher for our local farm team with the chief complaint of, "I can't raise my right arm and my right shoulder is really sore." Tommy stated that about a week ago, he was really trying to put one over the plate to finish the game when he felt like "something popped in my right shoulder. It really hurt, but it was strike three and I headed off to the locker room to ice my shoulder. I took a quick shower and when I tried to reach up to the top shelf of my locker to grab my wallet, I just couldn't do it. My arm just wouldn't work. I didn't say anything to anybody, because you know at my age. . ." as his voiced just trailed off. "But I figured with ice, Tylenol, and a couple days off, I would be right as rain. But here I am," he said with a weak smile. I asked if he had ever had anything like this before, and he shook his head and said, "No, just the usual aches and pains. The only time I ever missed a game was from some bad chili when we were taking a run through Texas. I had really hoped to finish out this season because it was going to be my last. I hope to find a coaching job because I love the game." I told Tommy I would do all I could for him and the first step was to figure out exactly what was going on with his shoulder. I asked Tommy how he was sleeping and he said pretty well, but every time he rolled over onto his right shoulder, he woke up. Tommy denied any fever or chills.

On physical examination, Tommy was afebrile. His respirations were 16 and his pulse was 64 and regular. His blood pressure was 118/82. His head, eyes, ears, nose, throat (HEENT) exam was normal, as was his cardiopulmonary examination. His thyroid was normal. His abdominal examination revealed no abnormal mass or organomegaly. There was a right lower quadrant scar that Tommy said was from an appendectomy when he was a kid. There was no costovertebral angle (CVA) tenderness. There was no peripheral edema. His low back examination was unremarkable. Visual inspection of the right shoulder revealed a small area of ecchymosis in the subacromial region. I asked Tommy to point with one finger to show me where it "hurts the most"

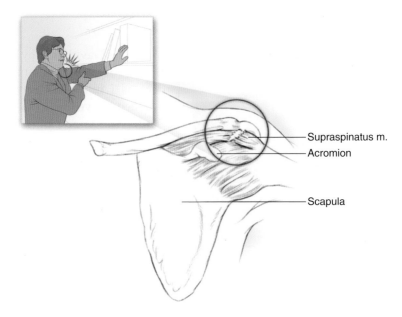

Fig. 8.1	Inability to elevate the arm above the level of the shoulder is the hallmark of rotator cuff dysfunction. (From Waldman SD. *Atlas of Common Pain Syndromes*. 4th ed. Philadelphia, PA: Elsevier; 2019 [Fig. 33.2].)

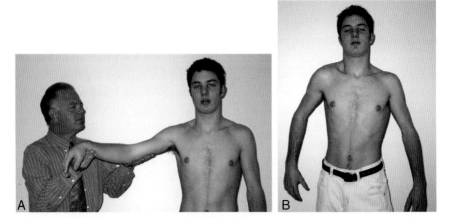

Fig. 8.2	(A) The drop arm test for complete rotator cuff tear. (B) A patient with a complete rotator cuff tear is unable to hold the arm in the abducted position, and it falls to the side. The patient often shrugs or hitches his shoulder forward to use the intact muscles of the rotator cuff and the deltoid to keep the arm in the abducted position. (From Waldman SD. *Atlas of Common Pain Syndromes*. 4th ed. Philadelphia, PA: Elsevier; 2019 [Fig. 33.3 A,B].)

and he pointed to the subacromial area but noted that what really worried him wasn't the pain, but his inability to raise his right arm above the level of his shoulder. I asked Tommy to abduct his left arm as high as he could, which he did without difficulty. I asked him to repeat the maneuver on the right and at about 80 degrees of abduction, he began to experience pain and was unable to abduct his arm much higher, so he elevated his shoulder to compensate (Fig. 8.1). The right shoulder was a little warm but did not appear to be infected. Tommy exhibited a positive drop arm test as well as a positive Moseley test (Fig. 8.2). Passive range of motion (ROM) of the right shoulder was normal. Tommy's left shoulder examination was normal, as was examination of his other major joints. A careful neurologic examination of the upper extremities revealed that there was no evidence of peripheral or entrapment neuropathy, and the deep tendon reflexes were normal. I told Tommy I was pretty sure I knew what was going on and we were going to get some tests to confirm it.

Key Clinical Points—What's Important and What's Not
THE HISTORY

- A history of the sudden onset of the inability to abduct the right arm above the level of the shoulder following pitching a baseball
- The history of a sudden pop in the shoulder at the time of the acute injury
- A history of continued pain in spite of conservative therapy
- No history of previous significant shoulder pain
- No fever of chills
- Sleep disturbance
- Difficulty abducting the affected right upper extremity

THE PHYSICAL EXAMINATION

- The patient is afebrile
- Palpation of right shoulder reveals tenderness in the subacromial region on the right
- The presence of mild ecchymosis in the subacromial region on the right
- The inability of the patient to actively abduct the right arm above the level of the shoulder
- Normal passive abduction of the right shoulder
- A positive drop arm test
- A positive Moseley test

OTHER FINDINGS OF NOTE

- Normal HEENT examination
- Normal cardiovascular examination
- Normal pulmonary examination

- Normal abdominal examination with a well-healed appendectomy scar noted
- No peripheral edema
- Normal upper extremity neurologic examination, motor and sensory examination
- Examination of other joints was normal

What Tests Would You Like to Order?

The following tests were ordered:
- Plain radiographs of the right shoulder, including anteroposterior (AP), lateral, axillary views
- Magnetic resonance imaging (MRI) of the right shoulder
- Ultrasound of the right shoulder with special attention to the rotator cuff

TEST RESULTS

The plain radiographs of the right shoulder revealed marked narrowing of the subacromial space secondary to proximal humeral head migration (Fig. 8.3).

The MRI revealed a full-thickness tear of the supraspinatus tendon as well as more chronic tendinopathy of the infraspinatus tendon, as evidenced by thickening and high signal intensity of the tendon (Fig. 8.4).

The ultrasound of the right shoulder revealed a complete tear of the supraspinatus tendon and fluid within the defect (Fig. 8.5).

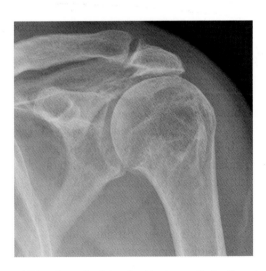

Fig. 8.3 Anteroposterior (AP) radiograph of the shoulder in a patient with a chronic rotator cuff tear. There is marked narrowing of the subacromial space secondary to proximal humeral head migration. (From Waldman SD, Campbell RSD. *Imaging of Pain*. Philadelphia, PA: Saunders; 2011 [Fig. 93.3].)

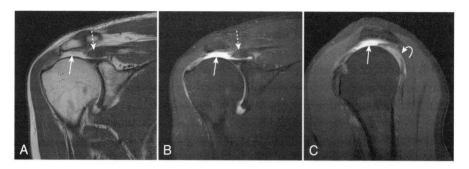

Fig. 8.4 Coronal oblique T1-weighted (T1W) (A) and T2W with fat suppression (FST2W) (B) magnetic resonance (MR) arthrogram images of a patient with a full-thickness tear of the supraspinatus tendon. The tendon defect is outlined by the high-signal intensity contrast medium *(white arrows)*, and the torn tendon end is visible medially *(broken white arrows)*. (C) The sagittal oblique FST2W MR image also demonstrates the tendon tear *(white arrow)*, and the infraspinatus tendon posteriorly *(curved arrow)* is thickened and has high signal intensity because of associated tendinopathy. (From Waldman SD, Campbell RSD. *Imaging of Pain*. Philadelphia, PA: Saunders; 2011 [Fig. 93.1].)

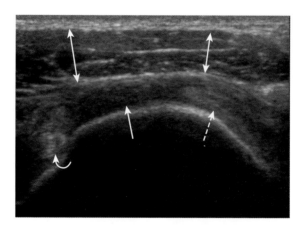

Fig. 8.5 Transverse ultrasound (US) image of a torn supraspinatus tendon. The tendon defect is filled by low-echo fluid *(white arrow);* it lies between the biceps tendon anteriorly *(curved arrow)* and the infraspinatus posteriorly *(broken white arrow)* and is deep to the deltoid muscle *(double-headed white arrows)*. (From Waldman SD, Campbell RSD. *Imaging of Pain*. Philadelphia, PA: Saunders; 2011 [Fig. 93.2].)

 Clinical Correlation—Putting It All Together

What is the diagnosis?
- Complete rotator cuff tear

The Science Behind the Diagnosis

ANATOMY OF THE ROTATOR CUFF

The rotator cuff, which is made up of the supraspinatus, infraspinatus, subscapularis, and teres minor muscles, provides shoulder movement and stability, along with the other associated ligaments and tendons (Fig. 8.6). All of the musculotendinous units of the rotator cuff are susceptible to tendinopathy and/or tear, with the supraspinatus and infraspinatus most often affected (Fig. 8.7). The rotator interval is a triangular space located between the supraspinatus and subscapularis tendons that provides easy sonographic access for ultrasound evaluation of the rotator cuff (Fig. 8.8). The base of the triangular space is formed by the coracoid process. The superior portion of the triangle is formed by the anterior margin of the supraspinatus muscle, with the inferior margin formed by the superior margin of the subscapularis muscle. The apex of the rotator interval triangle is the intertubercular groove. Within the triangular space of the rotator interval are the capsule of the glenohumeral joint, the coracohumeral ligament, the glenohumeral ligament, and the biceps tendon.

The supraspinatus and infraspinatus muscle tendons are particularly susceptible to the development of tendinitis for several reasons. First, the joint is subjected to many different repetitive motions. Second, the space in which the musculotendinous unit functions is restricted by the coracoacromial arch, thus making impingement likely with extreme joint movements. Third, the blood

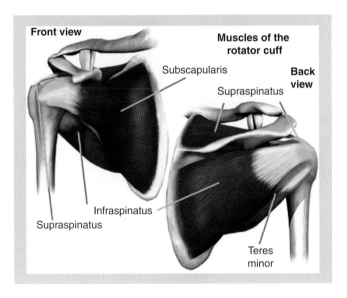

Fig. 8.6 The musculotendinous units of the rotator cuff. (From Vollans S, Ali A. Rotator cuff tears. *Surgery (Oxford)*. 2016:34(3):129–133 [Fig. 1].)

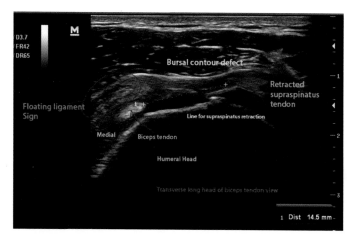

Fig. 8.7 Ultrasound image demonstrating full thickness tear of the supraspinatus tendon. Note the retracted suprapinatus tendon. (Courtesy Steven Waldman, MD.)

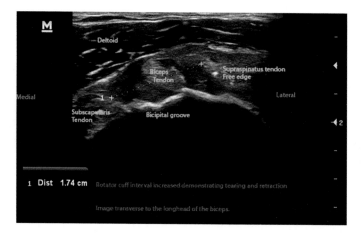

Fig. 8.8 The rotator interval demonstrating tearing and tendon retraction. (Courtesy Steven Waldman, MD.)

supply to the musculotendinous unit is poor, and this makes healing of microtrauma difficult. All these factors can contribute to tendinitis of one or more tendons of the shoulder joint. Calcium deposition around the tendon may occur if the inflammation continues, which complicates subsequent treatment. Bursitis often accompanies rotator cuff tears and may require specific treatment. In addition to pain, patients suffering from rotator cuff tear often experience a gradual reduction in functional ability because of decreasing shoulder ROM that makes simple everyday tasks such as combing one's hair, fastening a brassiere, or reaching overhead quite difficult. With continued disuse, muscle wasting may occur, and a frozen shoulder may develop.

CLINICAL CONSIDERATIONS

Rotator cuff tears are a common cause of shoulder pain and dysfunction. A rotator cuff tear frequently occurs after seemingly minor trauma to the musculotendinous unit of the shoulder. However, in most cases, the pathologic process responsible for the tear has been a long time in the making and is the result of ongoing tendinitis. The rotator cuff is made up of the subscapularis, supraspinatus, infraspinatus, and teres minor muscles and the associated tendons. The function of the rotator cuff is to rotate the arm and help provide shoulder joint stability along with the other muscles, tendons, and ligaments of the shoulder.

SIGNS AND SYMPTOMS

Patients presenting with rotator cuff tear frequently complain that they cannot raise the affected arm above the level of the shoulder without using the other arm to lift it (see Fig. 8.1). On physical examination, weakness on external rotation is noted if the infraspinatus is involved, and weakness on abduction above the level of the shoulder is evident if the supraspinatus is involved. Tenderness to palpation in the subacromial region is often present. Patients with partial rotator cuff tears lose the ability to reach overhead smoothly. Patients with complete tears exhibit anterior migration of the humeral head, as well as a complete inability to reach above the level of the shoulder. A positive drop arm test—the inability to hold the arm abducted at the level of the shoulder after the supported arm is released—is often seen with complete tears of the rotator cuff (see Fig. 8.2). The result of the Moseley test for rotator cuff tear is also positive; this test is performed by having the patient actively abduct the arm to 80 degrees and then adding gentle resistance, which forces the arm to drop if complete rotator cuff tear is present. Passive ROM of the shoulder is normal, but active ROM is limited. The pain of rotator cuff tear is constant and severe and is made worse with abduction and external rotation of the shoulder. Significant sleep disturbance is often reported. Patients may attempt to splint the inflamed subscapularis tendon by limiting medial rotation of the humerus.

TESTING

Plain radiographs are indicated in all patients who present with shoulder pain (see Fig. 8.3). Based on the patient's clinical presentation, additional testing may be indicated, including a complete blood count, erythrocyte sedimentation rate, and antinuclear antibody testing. MRI and ultrasound imaging of the shoulder are indicated if rotator cuff tendinopathy and/or tear is suspected (see Figs. 8.4, 8.7, and 8.8).

DIFFERENTIAL DIAGNOSIS

Because rotator cuff tears may occur after seemingly minor trauma, the diagnosis is often delayed. The tear may be either partial or complete, further confusing the diagnosis, although a careful physical examination can distinguish between the two. Tendinitis of the musculotendinous unit of the shoulder frequently coexists with bursitis of the associated bursae of the shoulder joint and creates additional pain and functional disability. This pain can cause the patient to splint the shoulder group, with resulting abnormal movement of the shoulder that puts additional stress on the rotator cuff and can lead to further trauma. With rotator cuff tears, passive ROM is normal, but active ROM is limited; with frozen shoulder, both passive ROM and active ROM are limited. Rotator cuff tear rarely occurs before age 40 years, except in cases of severe acute trauma to the shoulder.

TREATMENT

Initial treatment of the pain and functional disability associated with rotator cuff tear includes a combination of nonsteroidal antiinflammatory drugs (NSAIDs) or cyclooxygenase-2 (COX-2) inhibitors and physical therapy. Local application of heat and cold may also be beneficial. For patients who do not respond to these treatment modalities, the injection technique described here is a reasonable next step before surgical intervention.

Injection for rotator cuff tear is carried out by placing the patient in the supine position and preparing the skin overlying the superior shoulder, acromion, and distal clavicle with antiseptic solution. A sterile syringe containing 4 mL of 0.25% preservative-free bupivacaine and 40 mg methylprednisolone is attached to a 1.5-inch, 25-gauge needle using strict aseptic technique (Fig. 8.9). The lateral edge of the acromion is identified, and at the midpoint of the lateral edge, the injection site is identified. With a slightly cephalad trajectory, the needle is carefully advanced through the skin, subcutaneous tissues, and deltoid muscle beneath the acromion process. If bone is encountered, the needle is withdrawn into the subcutaneous tissues and is redirected slightly more inferiorly. After the needle is in place, the contents of the syringe are gently injected. Resistance to injection should be minimal unless calcification of the subacromial bursal sac is present. This calcification can be recognized as resistance to needle advancement, with an

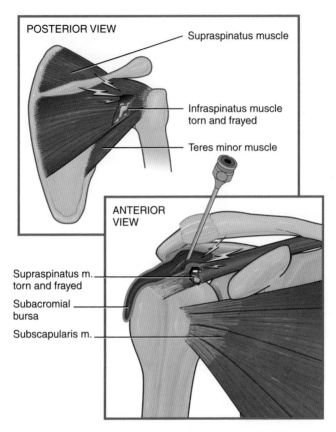

Fig. 8.9 Correct needle placement for injection of the rotator cuff. (From Waldman SD. *Atlas of Pain Management Injection Techniques*. 4th ed. St. Louis, MO: Elsevier; 2017 [Fig. 40.5].)

associated gritty feel. Significant calcific bursitis may ultimately require irrigation and barbotage or surgical excision to obtain complete relief of symptoms. After injection, the needle is removed, and a sterile pressure dressing and ice pack are applied to the injection site. Ultrasound needle guidance may be useful in those patients in whom anatomic landmarks are difficult to identify as well as to improve accuracy of needle placement. Recent clinical reports suggest that the injection of platelet-rich plasma and/or stem cells into the region of tendinopathy may aid in symptom relief and healing.

Physical modalities, including local heat and gentle ROM exercises, should be introduced several days after the patient undergoes injection. Transcutaneous nerve stimulation may also reduce pain control. Vigorous exercises should be avoided because they will exacerbate the patient's symptoms and may lead to complete tendon rupture.

HIGH-YIELD TAKEAWAYS

- The patient is afebrile, making an acute infectious etiology (e.g., septic arthritis) unlikely.
- The patient's symptomatology is the result of an acute throwing injury of the shoulder, and physical examination and testing should be focused on the identification of ligamentous injury and fracture.
- The patient's pain is localized to the insertion of the subacromial region.
- The patient's symptoms are unilateral and only involve one joint, which is more suggestive of a local process than a systemic polyarthropathy.
- Sleep disturbance is common and must be addressed concurrently with the patient's pain symptomatology.
- Plain radiographs will provide high-yield information regarding the bony contents of the joint, but ultrasound imaging and MRI will be more useful in identifying soft tissue pathology.
- Although the symptoms of acute rotator cuff tear often suddenly appear, the causes of tendinopathy are more chronic.

Suggested Readings

Allen H, Chan BY, Davis KW, et al. Overuse injuries of the shoulder. *Radiol Clin N Am.* 2019;58(5):898−909.

Cibulas A, Leyva A, Cibulas G, et al. Acute shoulder injury. *Radiol Clin N Am.* 2019;58 (5):883−898.

Netter FH. Shoulder (glenohumeral joint). In: *Atlas of Human Anatomy.* 4th ed. Philadelphia, PA: Saunders; 2008.

Waldman SD. Clinical correlates: functional anatomy of the shoulder. In: *Physical Diagnosis of Pain: An Atlas of Signs and Symptoms.* 3rd ed. Philadelphia, PA: Saunders; 2018.

Waldman SD. Rotator cuff disease. In: *Waldman's Comprehensive Atlas of Diagnostic Ultrasound of Painful Conditions.* Philadelphia, PA: Wolters Kluwer; 2016:186−195.

Waldman SD. Rotator cuff tear. In: Waldman SD, ed. *Atlas of Common Pain Syndromes.* 4th ed. Philadelphia, PA: Elsevier; 2019:129−133.

Waldman SD, ed. *Atlas of Pain Management Injection Techniques.* 4th ed. Philadelphia, PA: Saunders; 2018:94−98.

Waldman SD. Clinical correlates: diseases of the rotator cuff. In: *Physical Diagnosis of Pain: An Atlas of Signs and Symptoms.* 3rd ed. Philadelphia, PA: Elsevier; 2016:87−92.

Donald Harrison

A 67-Year-Old Male With
Acute-Onset Right Anterior
Shoulder Pain Associated With
an Audible Pop

- Learn the common causes of shoulder pain.
- Develop an understanding of the unique anatomy of the shoulder joint.
- Develop an understanding of the anatomy of the biceps tendon and biceps muscle.
- Understand the function of the biceps tendon.
- Develop an understanding of the causes of biceps tendon rupture.
- Develop an understanding of the various types of biceps tendon pathology.
- Learn the clinical presentation of biceps tendon rupture.
- Learn how to examine the biceps tendon.
- Learn how to use physical examination to identify pathology of the biceps tendon.
- Develop an understanding of the treatment options for biceps tendon rupture.

Donald Harrison

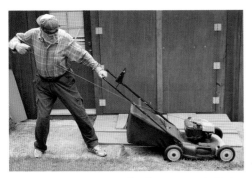

Donald Harrison is a 67-year-old retired postal worker with the chief complaint of, "My arm looks like Popeye The Sailor Man and I still can't start that gall darn lawn-mower." I laughed and said, "Donald, tell me exactly what happened." "My wife kept telling me to get a new lawn mower—you know, the one with an electric start. But my lawn mower was still plenty good. It just gets stubborn sometimes." "Okay," I said, "but tell me what happened to your arm." "That's what I am trying to tell you. Doc. Just hold your horses! I like to keep a nice yard, so I went out to mow it and the gol-darn lawn mower decided to get stubborn. I bet I pulled on that rope 15 times and it would cough a few times and then just die. The last time, I gave it a great big pull with all of my might and I heard this pop in my shoulder and it started hurting big time; and with all that, the gol-darn thing coughed a couple of times and died. I went inside to put some IcyHot on the front of my arm, so I takes my shirt off and I look in the mirror and I think my eyes are playing tricks on me. I have a big bruise on the top of my arm in front and it looks like I just ate a can of spinach—I looked just like Popeye. I knew there was going to be a lot of 'I told you sos' when Elizabeth—that's my wife—found out." I broke in and asked, "Donald, have your shoulder and upper arm been bothering you?" He shook his head no and said, "I may look like 10 miles of bad road, but I am as tough as an old boot." I laughed again and asked Donald how he was sleeping. He said that as long as he didn't lie on his bad arm, it was lights out and sweet dreams. Donald denied any fever or chills associated with his pain.

On physical examination, Donald was afebrile. His respirations were 18 and his pulse was 64 and regular. His blood pressure was 148/90. His head, eyes, ears, nose, throat (HEENT) exam was normal, as was his cardiopulmonary examination. He had a bunch of actinic keratoses on his face and the backs of his hands that would need attention sooner rather than later. His thyroid was normal. His abdominal examination revealed no abnormal mass or organomegaly. There was a right subcostal scar that Donald said was from having his gallstones removed. There was no costovertebral angle (CVA) tenderness. There was no peripheral edema. His low back examination was unremarkable. Visual inspection of the right shoulder revealed a large area of ecchymosis over the bicipital groove. I asked Donald to point with one finger to show me where it "hurts the most" and he pointed to the bicipital groove, but before I could go on, he pointed to the bulge in his anterior right arm just above the elbow and said, "Doc, let's

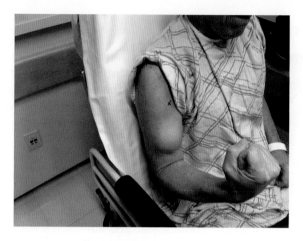

Fig. 9.1   Typical Popeye deformity seen with rupture of the long head of the biceps tendon. (From Virk MS, Cole BJ. Proximal biceps tendon and rotator cuff tears. *Clin Sports Med.* 2016;35(1):153–161.)

not worry about the pain. You need to tell me what the heck this is!" (Fig. 9.1). I said to Donald, "I know exactly what it is and I know exactly what to do about it, so I got this! Let me make sure nothing else is going on and then together we will map out a plan. I promise it will not involve eating any more spinach!" He laughed and said, "You're the doctor." I then asked Donald to place his hands behind his head and make a muscle like Popeye. As expected, the Ludington maneuver was positive (Fig. 9.2).

I noted that Donald was splinting his affected upper extremity by internally rotating his shoulder to move the biceps tendon from beneath the coracoacromial arch. He was tender over the right bicipital groove and his passive range of motion of upper extremity flexion at the elbow was completely normal, but it was obvious that active flexion on the right caused Donald some pain. I noted the large ecchymosis overlying the bicipital groove on the right, which certainly went along with my suspected diagnosis. Passive range of motion of the right shoulder was normal. Donald's left shoulder examination was normal, as was examination of his other major joints. A careful neurologic examination of the upper extremities revealed that there was no evidence of peripheral or entrapment neuropathy, and the deep tendon reflexes were normal. I told Donald that I was pretty sure that the lawn mower had got the best of him and he pulled on that starter rope one too many times and ruptured the long head of his biceps tendon. The Popeye bump was his biceps muscle bunched up in front of his elbow. I told him that I want to get a confirmatory test to ascertain the condition of the proximal tendon so we could better go in and sew it all back together.

Donald said, "You know, Doc (and you can't tell my Elizabeth), that gol-darn lawn mower wasn't being stubborn, it was out of gas!"

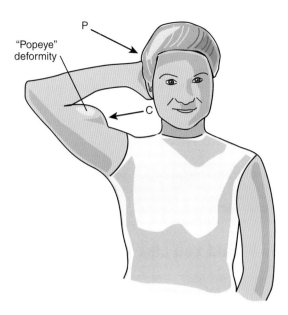

Fig. 9.2 The Ludington maneuver for ruptured long tendon of the biceps. *C*, Contraction of biceps; *P*, pressure applied. (From Waldman SD. *Atlas of Common Pain Syndromes*. 4th ed. Philadelphia, PA: Elsevier; 2019 [Fig. 31.4].)

Key Clinical Points—What's Important and What's Not

THE HISTORY

- A history of the sudden onset of the anterior upper arm pain with an associated cosmetic deformity
- The history of a sudden audible pop in the shoulder at the time of the acute injury
- A history of significant ecchymosis over the bicipital groove
- No history of previous significant shoulder pain
- No fever of chills
- Sleep disturbance

THE PHYSICAL EXAMINATION

- The patient is afebrile
- Palpation of right shoulder reveals tenderness over the bicipital groove on the right
- The presence of significant ecchymosis over the bicipital groove on the right
- Normal passive range of motion of the right shoulder
- Normal passive elbow flexion on the right
- A positive Ludington maneuver (see Fig. 9.2)

OTHER FINDINGS OF NOTE

- Normal HEENT examination
- Actinic keratosis over face and back of hands
- Normal cardiovascular examination
- Normal pulmonary examination
- Normal abdominal examination with a well-healed cholecystectomy scar noted
- No peripheral edema
- Normal upper extremity neurologic examination, motor and sensory examination
- Examination of other joints was normal

 ## What Tests Would You Like to Order?

The following tests were ordered:
- Magnetic resonance imaging (MRI) of the right shoulder to ascertain the condition of the proximal biceps tendon
- Ultrasound of the right shoulder with special attention to the proximal biceps tendon

TEST RESULTS

The MRI revealed extensive rotator cuff tendinopathy and rupture of the long head of the biceps tendon. The tendon sheath within the bicipital groove is filled by high signal intensity (SI) contrast, and no tendon is visible (Fig. 9.3, note *arrow*).

The ultrasound of the right biceps tendon revealed a complete tear of the biceps tendon with bunching of the biceps muscle on contraction (Fig. 9.4).

 ## Clinical Correlation—Putting It All Together

What is the diagnosis?
- Rupture of the long head of the biceps tendon

The Science Behind the Diagnosis

ANATOMY OF THE BICEPS TENDON

Along with the conjoined tendons of the rotator cuff, the bicipital muscle serves to stabilize the shoulder joint. The biceps muscle, which is named for its two heads, functions to supinate the forearm and flex the elbow joint (Fig. 9.5).

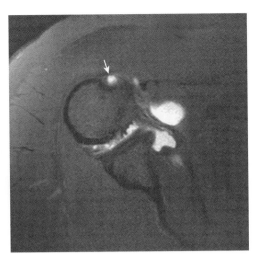

Fig. 9.3 Axial T1-weighted with fat suppression (FST1W) magnetic resonance (MR) arthrogram image of a patient with an extensive rotator cuff tear and rupture of the long head of biceps (LHB) tendon. The tendon sheath within the bicipital groove is filled by high signal intensity (SI) contrast, and no tendon is visible *(white arrow)*. (From Waldman SD, Campbell RSD. *Imaging of Pain*. Philadelphia, PA: Saunders; 2011 [Fig. 97.1].)

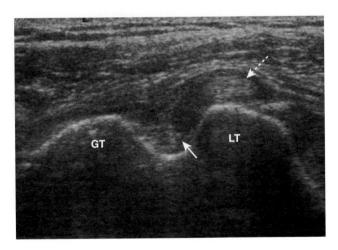

Fig. 9.4 Transverse US image of the proximal humerus demonstrating an empty bicipital groove *(white arrow)*. However, the long head of biceps tendon is subluxated medially and is clearly visible lying on the lesser tuberosity *(broken white arrow)*. When the tendon is dislocated more medially, it can be difficult to identify and can be mistaken for a tendon rupture. (From Waldman SD, Campbell RSD. *Imaging of Pain*. Philadelphia, PA: Saunders; 2011 [Fig. 97.3].)

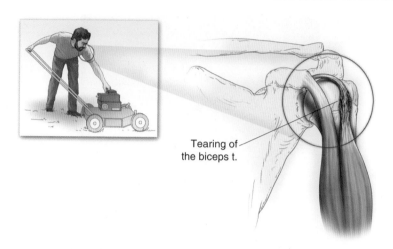

Tearing of
the biceps t.

Fig. 9.5 The onset of pain and functional disability associated with biceps tendon tear is generally acute, occurring after overuse or misuse of the shoulder joint, such as trying to start a recalcitrant lawn mower. (From Waldman SD. *Atlas of Common Pain Syndromes*. 4th ed. Philadelphia, PA: Elsevier; 2019 [Fig. 31.1].)

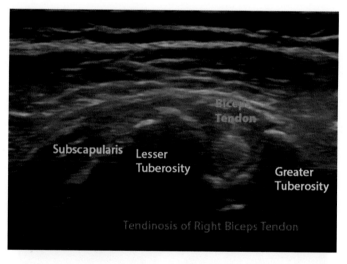

Fig. 9.6 Ultrasound image of the biceps tendon within the bicipital groove. Note the mild tendinosis of the tendon. (Courtesy Steven Waldman, MD.)

The long head finds its origin in the supraglenoid tubercle of the scapula, and the short head finds its origin from the tip of the coracoid process of the scapula. The long head exits the shoulder joint via the bicipital groove, where it is susceptible to trauma and the development of tendinitis (Figs. 9.6 and 9.7). The long

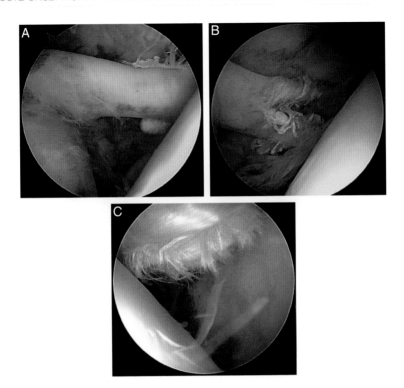

Fig. 9.7 Arthroscopic images of the long head of the biceps tendon as seen from the posterior portal showing synovitis (A), partial tear (B), and delamination (C) of the long head of the biceps, concomitant with rotator cuff tear. (From Waldman SD. *Atlas of Common Pain Syndromes*. 4th ed. Philadelphia, PA: Elsevier; 2019 [Fig. 31.2].)

head fuses with the short head in the middle portion of the upper arm, forming the belly of the biceps muscle. The insertion of the biceps muscle is into the posterior portion of the radial tuberosity. The biceps muscle is innervated by the musculocutaneous nerve, which arises from the lateral cord of the brachial plexus. The fibers of the musculocutaneous nerve are derived from C5, C6, and C7 nerve roots. The biceps musculotendinous unit is subjected to significant stress during functioning, and misuse or orveruse can result in inflammation and damage. If the damage remains untreated, the musculotendinous unit can rupture (see Figs. 9.3 and 9.4). This most commonly occurs with the long head of the biceps, but the short head and the distal tendinous insertion can also rupture (Fig. 9.8).

CLINICAL CONSIDERATIONS

The tendons of the long and short heads of the biceps are particularly susceptible to the development of tendinitis. Biceps tendon tear is usually

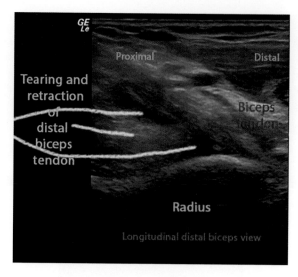

Fig. 9.8 Ultrasound image showing tearing of the distal biceps tendon at its insertion at the elbow. (Courtesy Steven Waldman, MD.)

caused at least partially by impingement on the tendons of the biceps at the coracoacromial arch. The onset of pain and functional disability associated with biceps tendon tear is generally acute, occurring after overuse or misuse of the shoulder joint, such as trying to start a recalcitrant lawn mower, practicing an overhead tennis serve, or performing an overaggressive follow-through when driving golf balls. More common in men, proximal rupture of the tendon of the long head of the biceps tendon accounts for more than 97% of biceps tendon ruptures; ruptures of the distal portion of the biceps tendon occur less than 3% of the time. Rupture of the long head of the biceps tendon generally occurs in the fourth to sixth decades, but it can occur in younger age groups involved in high-risk activities such as snowboarding. The biceps muscle and tendons are intimately involved in shoulder and upper extremity function and are susceptible to trauma and to wear and tear (see Fig. 9.7). If the damage is severe enough, the tendon of the long head of the biceps can rupture, leaving the patient with a telltale "Popeye" biceps (named after the cartoon character) (see Fig. 9.1). This deformity can be accentuated by having the patient perform a Ludington maneuver (i.e., placing the hands behind the head and flexing the biceps muscle) (see Fig. 9.2).

SIGNS AND SYMPTOMS

In most patients, the pain of biceps tendon tear occurs acutely and is accompanied by a pop or snapping sound. The pain is constant and severe and is localized in the anterior shoulder over the bicipital groove (Fig. 9.9).

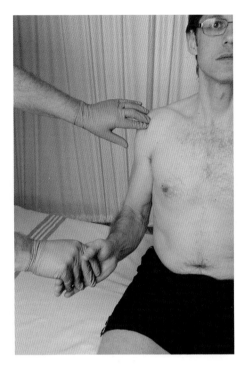

Fig. 9.9 Palpation of the bicipital groove. (Courtesy Steven Waldman, MD.)

Ecchymosis may be present if the trauma is acute and severe. Significant sleep disturbance is often reported. Patients with a partial tendon tear and significant tendinitis may attempt to splint the affected shoulder by internal rotation of the humerus, which moves the biceps tendon from beneath the coracoacromial arch. Patients with biceps tendon tear have a positive Ludington test result, as described earlier. Bursitis and tendinitis often accompany biceps tendon tear (Fig. 9.10). Occasionally, patients with acute tear of the long tendon of the biceps may experience only vague discomfort and seek medical attention only because of the cosmetic abnormality of the retracted biceps tendon and muscle. Occasionally, without treatment, frozen shoulder may develop.

TESTING

Magnetic resonance imaging of the shoulder is indicated if tendinopathy or tear of the biceps tendon is suspected. Ultrasound imaging may also help further delineate the pathology responsible for the patient's pain and functional disability (Fig. 9.11). The injection technique described later serves as both a diagnostic and a therapeutic maneuver.

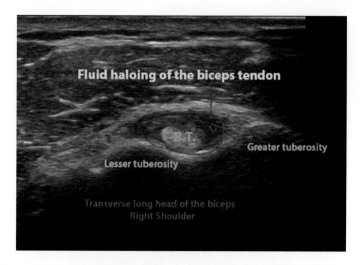

Fig. 9.10 Transverse ultrasound image of the biceps tendon within the bicipital groove with haloing around the tendon secondary to bicipital tendinitis. (Courtesy Steven Waldman, MD.)

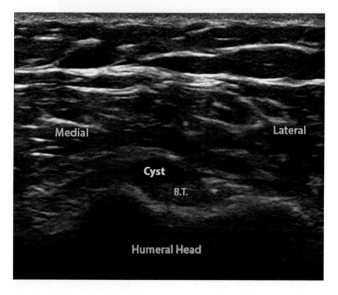

Fig. 9.11 Transverse ultrasound image of the biceps tendon, demonstrating a cyst impinging on the biceps tendon. (Courtesy Steven Waldman, MD.)

DIFFERENTIAL DIAGNOSIS

Biceps tendon tear is usually a straightforward clinical diagnosis. However, coexisting bursitis or tendinitis of the shoulder from overuse or misuse may confuse the diagnosis. Occasionally, partial rotator cuff tear can be mistaken for biceps tendon tear. In some clinical situations, consideration should be given to primary or secondary tumors involving the shoulder, superior sulcus of the lung, or proximal humerus. The pain of acute herpes zoster, which occurs before eruption of a vesicular rash, can also mimic biceps tendon tear.

TREATMENT

Initial treatment of the pain and functional disability associated with biceps tendon tear includes a combination of nonsteroidal antiinflammatory drugs (NSAIDs) or cyclooxygenase-2 (COX-2) inhibitors and physical therapy. Local application of heat and cold may also be beneficial. For patients who do not respond to these treatment modalities and who appear to have significant local pain in the region of the bicipital groove, injection with local anesthetic and steroid is a reasonable next step.

Injection for biceps tendon tear is carried out by placing the patient in the supine position with the arm externally rotated approximately 45 degrees. The coracoid process is identified anteriorly. Just lateral to the coracoid process is the lesser tuberosity, which can be more easily palpated as the arm is passively rotated. The point overlying the tuberosity is marked with a sterile marker. The skin overlying the anterior shoulder is prepared with antiseptic solution. A sterile syringe containing 1 mL of 0.25% preservative-free bupivacaine and 40 mg methylprednisolone is attached to a 1.5-inch, 25-gauge needle using strict aseptic technique. The previously marked point is palpated, and the insertion of the biceps tendon is reidentified with the gloved finger. Ultrasound guidance may help with identification of these anatomic structures (Fig. 9.12). The needle is carefully advanced at this point through the skin, subcutaneous tissues,

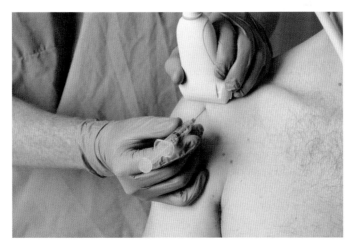

Fig. 9.12 Proper needle position for injection of the biceps tendon at the bicipital groove. (Courtesy Steven Waldman, MD.)

and underlying tendon until it impinges on bone. The needle is then withdrawn 1 to 2 mm out of the periosteum of the humerus, and the contents of the syringe are gently injected. Slight resistance to injection should be felt. If no resistance is encountered, either the needle tip is in the joint space itself or the tendon is ruptured. If resistance is significant, the needle tip is probably in the substance of a ligament or tendon and should be advanced or withdrawn slightly until the injection can proceed without significant resistance. The needle is then removed, and a sterile pressure dressing and ice pack are applied to the injection site. Physical modalities, including local heat and gentle range of motion exercises, should be introduced several days after the patient undergoes injection. Vigorous exercises should be avoided, because they will exacerbate the patient's symptoms. Occasionally, surgical repair of the tendon is undertaken if the patient is experiencing significant functional disability or is unhappy with the cosmetic defect resulting from the retracted tendon and muscle.

HIGH-YIELD TAKEAWAYS

- The patient is afebrile, making an acute infectious etiology (e.g., septic arthritis) unlikely.
- The patient's symptomatology is the result of an acute injury to the proximal biceps tendon, although damage and inflammation of the tendon over time may predispose the tendon to rupture.
- Physical examination and testing should be focused on the identification of causes of the patient's pain and functional disability.
- The patient's pain is localized to the insertion of the bicipital groove.
- Rupture of the proximal biceps tendon causes a classic Popeye deformity of the biceps muscle as it bunches due to unopposed contraction of its intact distal musculotendinous units.
- The patient's symptoms are unilateral and only involve one joint, which is more suggestive of a local process than a systemic polyarthropathy.
- Sleep disturbance is common and must be addressed concurrently with the patient's pain symptomatology.
- Plain radiographs will provide high-yield information regarding the bony contents of the joint, but ultrasound imaging and MRI will be more useful in identifying soft tissue pathology.
- Although the symptoms of acute rupture of the proximal biceps tendon often suddenly appear, the causes of tendinopathy are more chronic in nature.
- Less commonly, the distal biceps tendon may rupture just above its insertion on the radius at the elbow.

Suggested Readings

MacInnes SJ, Crawford LA, Shahane SA. Disorders of the biceps and triceps tendons at the elbow. *Orthop Trauma*. 2016;30(4):346–354.

McFarland EG, Borade A. Examination of the biceps tendon. *Clin Sports Med*. 2016;35 (1):29–45.

Thomas JR, Lawton JN. Biceps and triceps ruptures in athletes. *Hand Clin*. 2017;33 (1):35–46.

Virk MS, Cole BJ. Proximal biceps tendon and rotator cuff tears. *Clin Sports Med*. 2016;35(1):153–161.

Waldman SD. Bicipital tendinitis. In: *Atlas of Pain Management Injection Techniques*. 4th ed. Philadelphia, PA: Elsevier; 2017:114–117.

Waldman SD. The biceps tendon. In: *Pain Review*. 2nd ed. Philadelphia, PA: Elsevier; 2017:91–92.

Waldman SD, Campbell RSD. Biceps tendinopathy. In: *Imaging of Pain*. Philadelphia, PA: Saunders; 2011:245–246.

Mai Davika

A 19-Year-Old Female With Deep-Aching Shoulder Pain With Associated Weakness

- Learn the common causes of shoulder pain.
- Learn the common causes of shoulder weakness.
- Develop an understanding of the unique anatomy of the shoulder joint.
- Develop an understanding of the anatomy of the suprascapular nerve and surrounding structures.
- Develop an understanding of the causes of suprascapular nerve entrapment.
- Develop an understanding of the differential diagnosis of suprascapular nerve entrapment.
- Learn the clinical presentation of suprascapular nerve entrapment.
- Learn how to examine the shoulder.
- Learn how to use physical examination to identify suprascapular nerve entrapment.
- Develop an understanding of the treatment options for suprascapular nerve entrapment.

Mai Davika

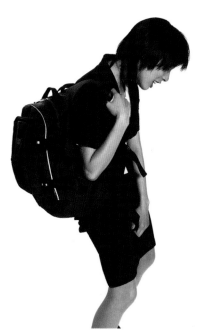

Mai Davika is a 19-year-old college student with the chief complaint of, "Something is wrong with my right shoulder. It hurts and feels weak." Mai stated that over the past 6 to 8 weeks, she began noticing that it was becoming more difficult to brush her hair. She also noticed that she was experiencing a deep, dull ache in the posterior aspect of her right shoulder, especially after carrying her backpack to class. More recently, Mai began to have difficulty reaching across her chest when reaching for her seat belt. I asked Mai if she had ever experienced anything like this in the past and she said no. I asked whether she had switched backpacks or was carrying more books than usual and she admitted that this semester, she is carrying more books than during past semesters and that she was also bringing her lunch and a couple of bottles of water so she could remain on campus and study. She denied any fever, chills, or other constitutional symptoms. I asked Mai what made her pain better and she said resting her shoulder and Motrin. I asked if she had tried ice or heat and she said that she tried a heating pad but thought it made the shoulder worse. She denied significant sleep disturbance

I asked Mai about any antecedent shoulder trauma and she just shook her head no. This time, the pain just wouldn't go away in spite of using the Motrin and a heating pad. Mai said that she felt that her shoulder was kind of weak, that it just didn't feel right. I asked Mai what made her pain worse and she said that her pain was worst when she looked to the left and reached across her chest to grab her seat belt.

I asked Mai to point with one finger to show me where it hurt the most. She pointed to the top of the right scapula and posterior aspect of the right shoulder and said, "It's really the whole back of my shoulder that hurts and it just feels kind of weak."

On physical examination, Mai was afebrile. Her respirations were 16 and her pulse was 68 and regular. Her blood pressure was 118/70. Mai's head, eyes, ears, nose, throat (HEENT) exam was normal, as was her cardiopulmonary examination. Her thyroid was normal. Her abdominal examination revealed no abnormal mass or organomegaly. There was no costovertebral angle (CVA) tenderness. There was no peripheral edema. Her low back examination was unremarkable. Visual inspection of the right shoulder revealed slight atrophy of the infraspinatus muscle. There was marked tenderness to palpation of the area overlying the right suprascapular notch.

Movement of the shoulder and especially abduction of the right scapula when having Mai reach across her chest reproduced Mai's pain complaint. Having Mai look to the left while her right shoulder was abducted also exacerbated the pain. The left shoulder examination was normal, as was examination of her other major joints. A careful neurologic examination of the upper extremities revealed that there was no evidence of peripheral neuropathy, but there was weakness of the infraspinatus muscle. Deep tendon reflexes were normal.

Key Clinical Points—What's Important and What's Not

THE HISTORY

- A history of acute trauma
- No history of previous significant shoulder pain
- No fever of chills
- Gradual onset of shoulder pain following carrying a backpack that was heavier than usual
- Exacerbation of pain when abducting the scapula and reaching across the chest
- Exacerbation of pain when looking toward the contralateral shoulder when reaching across the chest

THE PHYSICAL EXAMINATION

- The patient is afebrile
- Point tenderness to palpation of the area over the right suprascapular notch
- Mild atrophy of the infraspinatus muscle
- Mild weakness of the infraspinatus muscle
- No evidence of infection
- Pain on range of motion of the right shoulder, especially abduction of the right scapula when reaching across the chest

OTHER FINDINGS OF NOTE

- Normal HEENT examination
- Normal cardiovascular examination

- Normal pulmonary examination
- Normal abdominal examination
- No peripheral edema
- Normal upper extremity neurologic examination, motor and sensory examination with exception of slight weakness of the right infraspinatus muscle
- Examination of other joints other than the right shoulder were normal

 ## What Tests Would You Like to Order?

The following tests were ordered:
- Plain radiographs of the right shoulder
- Ultrasound of the right shoulder with special attention to the suprascapular notch
- Magnetic resonance imaging (MRI) of the right shoulder
- Electromyography (EMG) and nerve conduction velocity testing of the right brachial plexus, upper extremity, with special attention to the suprascapular nerve

TEST RESULTS

The plain radiographs of the right shoulder were normal.

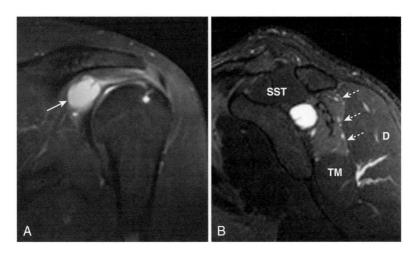

Fig. 10.1 (A) Coronal oblique T2-weighted (T2W) with fat suppression (FST2W) magnetic resonance (MR) image of a patient with a high-signal intensity paralabral cyst in the spinoglenoid notch *(white arrow)*. (B) A sagittal oblique FST2W MR image shows the cyst. There is also high SI within the infraspinatus muscle belly *(broken white arrows)* in comparison with the supraspinatus, teres minor, and deltoid muscle bellies. This finding indicates muscle denervation edema due to compression of the suprascapular nerve by the cyst. *D,* Deltoid; *SST,* supraspinatus; *TM,* teres minor. (From Waldman SD, Campbell RSD. *Imaging of Pain*. Philadelphia, PA: Saunders; 2011 [Fig. 101.1].)

Ultrasound examination of the right shoulder was unremarkable other than some atrophy of the infraspinatus muscle. Evaluation of the right suprascapular notch and its contents revealed a paralabral cyst impinging into the supracapular notch.

MRI scan of the right shoulder revealed a paralabral cyst in the notch as well as muscle denervation of the infraspinatus muscle (Fig. 10.1).

EMG and nerve conduction testing of the right brachial plexus and upper extremity revealed a normal examination of the right brachial plexus and no evidence of a peripheral neuropathy but denervation of the infraspinatus muscle.

Clinical Correlation—Putting It All Together

What is the diagnosis?
- Suprascapular nerve entrapment

The Science Behind the Diagnosis

ANATOMY

The suprascapular nerve is formed from fibers originating from the C5 and C6 nerve roots of the brachial plexus with some contribution of fibers from the C4 root in most patients. The nerve passes inferiorly and posteriorly from the brachial plexus to pass underneath the coracoclavicular ligament through the suprascapular notch. The suprascapular artery and vein accompany the nerve through the suprascapular notch (Figs. 10.2 and 10.3). The suprascapular nerve provides much of the sensory innervation to the shoulder joint and provides motor innervation to two of the muscles of the rotator cuff and the supraspinatus and infraspinatus muscles.

CLINICAL SYNDROME

Suprascapular nerve entrapment is an uncommon cause of shoulder pain that is being encountered more frequently in clinical practice with the increasing use of backpacks instead of briefcases (Fig. 10.4). Suprascapular nerve entrapment syndrome is caused by compression of the suprascapular nerve as it passes through the suprascapular notch. The most common causes of compression of the suprascapular nerve at this anatomic location include the prolonged wearing of heavy backpacks and direct blows to the nerve such as occur in football injuries and in falls from trampolines. Suprascapular nerve entrapment syndrome also is seen in baseball pitchers and quarterbacks.

This entrapment neuropathy manifests most commonly as a severe, deep, aching pain that radiates from the top of the scapula to the ipsilateral shoulder.

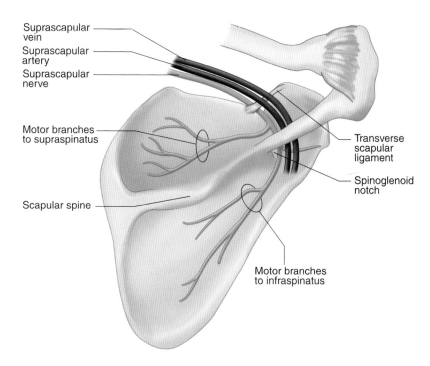

Fig. 10.2   Anatomy of the suprascapular nerve. (From Erickson B, Romeo A. *Operative Techniques: Shoulder and Elbow Surgery*. 2nd ed. Philadelphia, PA: Elsevier; 2019 [Fig. 43.3].)

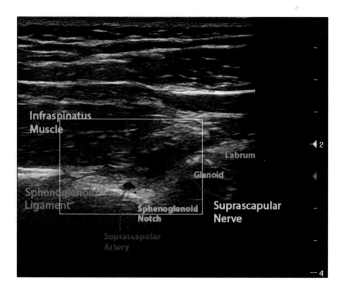

Fig. 10.3   Color Doppler image demonstrating the relationship between the suprascapular nerve and artery as they patch through the suprascapular notch. (Courtesy Steven Waldman, MD.)

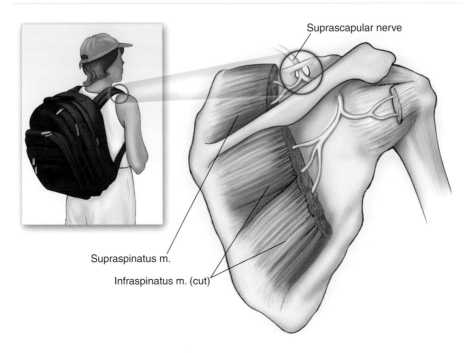

Fig. 10.4   Suprascapular nerve entrapment is caused by compression of the suprascapular nerve as it passes through the suprascapular notch. *m*, Muscle. (From Waldman SD. *Atlas of Uncommon Pain Syndromes*. 3rd ed. Philadelphia, PA: Saunders; 2014 [Fig. 34.1].)

Tenderness over the suprascapular notch is usually present. Shoulder movement, especially reaching across the chest, may increase the pain. If left untreated, weakness and atrophy of the supraspinatus and infraspinatus muscles occur.

SIGNS AND SYMPTOMS

The most important finding in patients with suprascapular nerve entrapment is weakness of the supraspinatus and infraspinatus muscles. This weakness manifests itself as weakness of abduction and external rotation of the ipsilateral shoulder. With significant compromise of the suprascapular nerve, atrophy of the infraspinatus muscle is apparent as it lies superficially. The pain of suprascapular nerve entrapment can be exacerbated by abducting the ipsilateral scapula by reaching across the chest and simultaneously rotating the neck away from the involved shoulder. Tenderness to palpation of the suprascapular notch is often present.

TESTING

Electromyography helps to distinguish cervical radiculopathy and Parsonage-Turner syndrome from suprascapular nerve entrapment syndrome. Plain

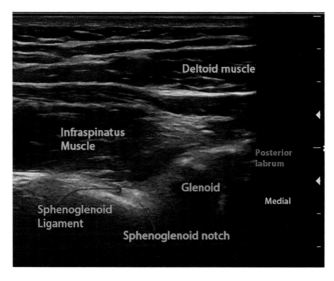

Fig. 10.5 Ultrasound imaging may also aid in the identification of causes of shoulder pain entrapment. (Courtesy Steven Waldman, MD.)

TABLE 10.1 ■ Differential Diagnosis of Suprascapular Nerve Entrapment

- Brachial plexopathy
- Parsonage-Turner syndrome
- Bursitis
- Tendinitis
- Shoulder arthritis
- Rotator cuff arthropathy
- Impingement syndromes
- Primary tumors of the shoulder
- Metastatic tumors to the shoulder

radiographs are indicated in all patients who present with suprascapular nerve entrapment syndrome to rule out occult bony pathology. Ultrasound imaging may also aid in the identification of this uncommon cause of shoulder pain (Fig. 10.5). Based on the patient's clinical presentation, additional testing, including complete blood cell count, uric acid level, erythrocyte sedimentation rate, and antinuclear antibody testing, may be indicated. MRI of the shoulder is indicated if a primary joint pathologic process or space-occupying lesion is suspected. The injection technique described here is a diagnostic and therapeutic maneuver.

DIFFERENTIAL DIAGNOSIS

Suprascapular nerve entrapment syndrome is often misdiagnosed as bursitis, tendinitis, or arthritis of the shoulder (Table 10.1). Cervical radiculopathy of the

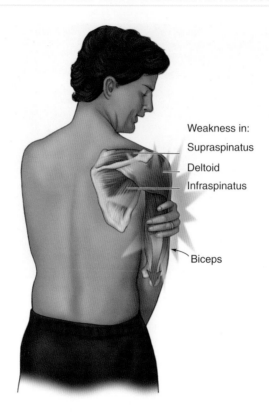

Weakness in:
Supraspinatus
Deltoid
Infraspinatus

Biceps

Fig. 10.6 The pain of Parsonage-Turner syndrome involves the shoulder and upper arm, preceding the onset of muscle weakness by hours to days. (From Waldman SD. *Atlas of Uncommon Pain Syndromes.* 3rd ed. Philadelphia, PA: Saunders; 2014 [Fig. 24.1].)

C5 nerve root also may mimic the clinical presentation of suprascapular nerve entrapment syndrome. Parsonage-Turner syndrome, also known as idiopathic brachial neuritis, may manifest as sudden onset of shoulder pain and can be confused with suprascapular nerve entrapment (Fig. 10.6). Tumor involving the superior scapular nerve, shoulder, or both, also should be considered in the differential diagnosis of suprascapular nerve entrapment syndrome.

TREATMENT

Nonsteroidal antiinflammatory drugs (NSAIDs) or cyclooxygenase-2 (COX-2) inhibitors represent a reasonable first step in the treatment of suprascapular nerve entrapment syndrome. The use of tricyclic antidepressants such as nortriptyline at a single bedtime dose of 25 mg, titrating upward as side effects allow, also is useful, especially if sleep disturbance also is present. Avoidance of repetitive trauma thought to be contributing to this entrapment neuropathy also

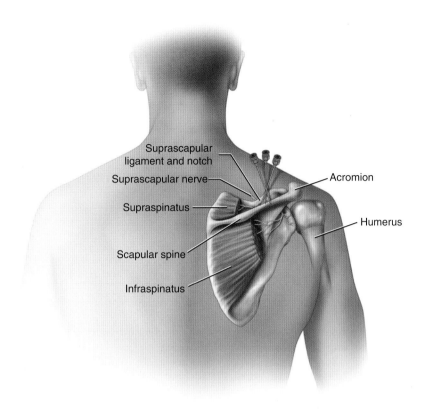

Fig. 10.7   Injection of the suprascapular nerve. (From Waldman SD. *Atlas of Pain Management Injection Techniques*. 4th ed. St. Louis, MO: Elsevier; 2017 [Fig. 41.6].)

is important, especially in professional athletes. If these maneuvers fail to produce rapid symptomatic relief, injection of the suprascapular nerve with local anesthetic and steroid is a reasonable next step (Fig. 10.7). If symptoms persist, surgical exploration and release of the suprascapular nerve are indicated.

H I G H - Y I E L D   T A K E A W A Y S

- The patient is afebrile, making an acute infectious etiology (e.g., septic arthritis) unlikely.
- The patient's symptomatology is thought to be the result of carrying an overly heavy backpack.

(Continued)

- Physical examination and testing should be focused on the identification of weakness of the supraspinatus and infraspinatus muscles.
- The patient has point tenderness over the suprascapular notch.
- The patient's symptoms are unilateral and only involve one joint, which is more suggestive of a local process than a systemic polyarthropathy.
- The patient has infraspinatus muscle atrophy and weakness.
- Plain radiographs will provide high-yield information regarding the bony contents of the joint, but ultrasound imaging and MRI will be more useful in identifying soft tissue pathology.
- Electromyography and nerve conduction velocity testing will help delineate the location and degree of nerve compromise.

Suggested Readings

Fehrman DA, Orwin JF, Jennings RM. Suprascapular nerve entrapment by ganglion cysts: a report of six cases with arthroscopic findings and review of the literature. *Arthroscopy*. 1995;11:727–734.

Moore TP, Hunter RE. Suprascapular nerve entrapment. *Oper Tech Sports Med*. 1996;4:8–14.

Toussaint CP, Zager EL. What's new in common upper extremity entrapment neuropathies. *Neurosurg Clin North Am*. 2008;19:573–581.

Waldman SD. Suprascapular nerve entrapment. In: Waldman SD, ed. *Atlas of Uncommon Pain Syndromes*. 3rd ed. Philadelphia, PA: W.B. Saunders; 2014:96–98.

Waldman SD. Suprascapular nerve entrapment and compression. In: Waldman SD, ed. *Waldman's Comprehensive Atlas of Diagnostic Ultrasound of Painful Conditions*. Philadelphia, PA: Wolters Kluwer; 2016:228–234.

Waldman SD. Ultrasound guided suprascapular nerve block. In: Waldman SD, ed. *Waldman's Comprehensive Atlas of Ultrasound Guided Pain Management Injection Techniques*. Philadelphia, PA: Wolters Kluwer; 2014:281–265.

Waldman SD. Suprascapular nerve block. In: Waldman SD, ed. *Pain Review*. Philadelphia, PA: Saunders; 2009:439–440.

Waldman SD. Suprascapular nerve entrapment. In: Waldman SD, Campbell RSD, eds. *Imaging of Pain*. Philadelphia, PA: W.B. Saunders; 2011:257–258.

Joy Kinder

A 25-Year-Old Female With Lateral Elbow Pain

- Learn the common causes of elbow pain.
- Develop an understanding of the unique anatomy of the elbow joint.
- Develop an understanding of the anatomy of the lateral epicondyle and the common extensor tendon.
- Develop an understanding of the causes of tennis elbow.
- Develop an understanding of the differential diagnosis of tennis elbow.
- Learn the clinical presentation of tennis elbow.
- Learn how to examine the elbow.
- Learn how to use physical examination to identify tennis elbow.
- Develop an understanding of the treatment options for tennis elbow.

Joy Kinder

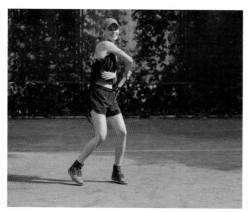

Joy Kinder is a 25-year-old PACU nurse with the chief complaint of "right elbow pain." Joy stated that over the past 4 or 5 weeks, she began noticing that her right elbow was becoming more and more painful. Joy stated that the pain started after she played in a weekend tennis match at the local country club. She said that she was playing with a new tennis racquet that may have been just a bit too heavy for her. She noted that after losing a close match in the finals, the outside of her right elbow was hurting. In spite of icing her elbow and taking naproxen, the pain continued to get worse. "Doctor, I don't mean to sound like a wimp, but I can barely lift my mug of coffee in the morning. The other thing that is really worrying me is that I feel like my grip is weak. I tried to go out and hit a few against the backboard, but I just couldn't hold the racquet." I asked Joy if she had any numbness associated with her pain and she just shook her head.

She denied any fever, chills, or other constitutional symptoms. I asked Joy what made her pain better and she said that maybe resting her elbow and taking Motrin helped. She denied significant sleep disturbance.

I asked Joy about any antecedent elbow trauma and she just shook her head no. She volunteered, "Doctor, this time the pain just wouldn't go away in spite of taking Advil and using a heating pad." Joy went on to say that she felt that her elbow was kind of weak and that it just didn't feel right.

I asked Joy to point with one finger to show me where it hurt the most. She pointed to the lateral epicondyle of the right elbow. "It really hurts all around this bone."

On physical examination, Joy was afebrile. Her respirations were 16 and her pulse was 72 and regular. Her blood pressure was 120/70. Joy's head, eyes, ears, nose, throat (HEENT) exam was normal as was her cardiopulmonary examination. Her thyroid was normal. Her abdominal examination revealed no abnormal mass or organomegaly. There was no costovertebral angel (CVA) tenderness. There was no peripheral edema. Her low back examination was unremarkable. Visual inspection of the right elbow revealed that the elbow was a little swollen. Palpation of the elbow revealed that the lateral aspect was a little warm. There was marked tenderness to palpation of the area overlying the right lateral epicondyle of the elbow. Palpation of the right forearm over the radial

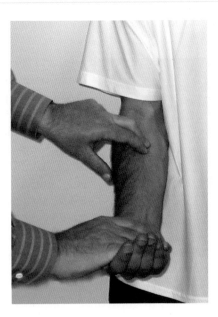

Fig. 11.1 Palpation of the radial nerve in the forearm to diagnosis radial tunnel syndrome. (Courtesy Steven Waldman, MD.)

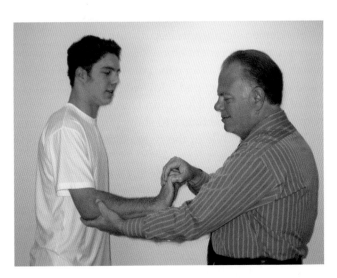

Fig. 11.2 The tennis elbow test is performed by stabilizing the patient's forearm and then having the patient clench the fist and actively extend the wrist. The examiner then attempts to force the wrist into flexion. Sudden, severe pain is highly suggestive of tennis elbow. (From Waldman SD. *Atlas of Common Pain Syndromes*. 4th ed. Philadelphia, PA: Elsevier; 2019 [Fig. 38.2].)

nerve did not reproduce Joy's pain (Fig. 11.1). Joy's tennis elbow test was markedly positive on the right (Fig. 11.2).

The left elbow examination was normal, as was examination of her other major joints. A careful neurologic examination of the upper extremities revealed that there was no evidence of peripheral neuropathy or entrapment neuropathy. Deep tendon reflexes were normal.

Key Clinical Points—What's Important and What's Not

THE HISTORY

- A history of onset of right lateral elbow pain after playing in a tennis tournament
- No history of previous significant elbow pain
- Weak grip strength
- No fever of chills
- Exacerbation of pain when lifting a coffee cup

THE PHYSICAL EXAMINATION

- The patient is afebrile
- Point tenderness to palpation of the area over the right lateral epicondyle
- No evidence of entrapment neuropathy
- Warmth and slight swelling over the right lateral epicondyle of the elbow
- Positive tennis elbow test
- No pain to palpation of the radial nerve in the forearm
- No evidence of infection

OTHER FINDINGS OF NOTE

- Normal HEENT examination
- Normal cardiovascular examination
- Normal pulmonary examination
- Normal abdominal examination
- No peripheral edema
- Normal upper extremity neurologic examination, motor and sensory examination
- Examination of other joints other than the right elbow were normal

 What Tests Would You Like to Order?

The following tests were ordered:
- Plain radiographs of the right elbow

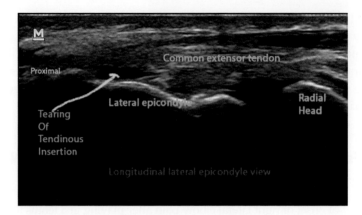

Fig. 11.3 Longitudinal ultrasound image of tennis elbow. (Courtesy Steven Waldman, MD.)

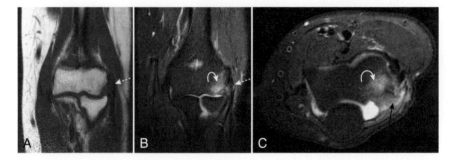

Fig. 11.4 Coronal photon density (A) and fat suppressed T2-weighted (FST2W) (B) magnetic reso-nance (MR) images of a patient with tennis elbow. There are thickening and increased signal intensity within the common extensor tendon *(broken white arrow)* along with associated underlying bone marrow edema *(curved arrow)*. (C) The bone marrow is also seen on the axial FST2W MR image *(curved arrow)*, and the soft tissue thickening and increased signal intensity posterior to the extensor tendon probably reflect associated soft tissue impingement *(black arrow)*. (From Waldman SD, Campbell RSD. *Imaging of Pain*. Philadelphia, PA: Saunders; 2011 [Fig. 103.2].)

- Ultrasound of the right elbow
- Magnetic resonance imaging (MRI) of the right elbow

TEST RESULTS

The plain radiographs of the right elbow were normal.

Ultrasound examination of the right elbow revealed tearing of the insertion of the common extensor tendon (Fig. 11.3).

MRI scan of the right elbow revealed thickening and increased signal intensity of the common extensor tendon as well as bone marrow edema of the lateral epicondyle (Fig. 11.4).

Clinical Correlation—Putting It All Together

What is the diagnosis?
- Tennis elbow (lateral epicondylitis)

The Science Behind the Diagnosis
ANATOMY

The most common nidus of pain from tennis elbow is the bony origin of the extensor tendon of the extensor carpi radialis brevis at the anterior facet of the lateral epicondyle (Fig. 11.5). Less commonly, tennis elbow pain can originate from the origin of the extensor carpi radialis longus at the supracondylar crest or, rarely, more distally at the point where the extensor carpi radialis brevis overlies the radial head. As mentioned earlier, bursitis may accompany tennis elbow. The olecranon bursa lies in the posterior aspect of the elbow joint and may also

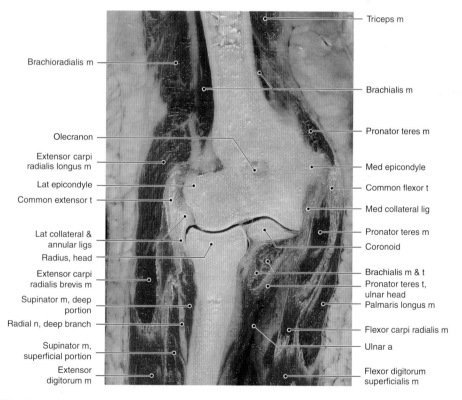

Fig. 11.5 Anatomy of the lateral epicondyle and common extensor tendon. (From Waldman SD, Bloch J. *Pain Management*. Philadelphia, PA: Saunders; 2007 [Fig. 63.1].)

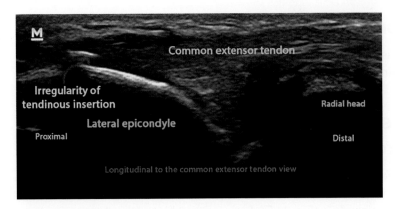

Fig. 11.6 Ultrasound examination demonstrating tendinopathy consistent with chronic lateral epicondylitis. (Courtesy Steven Waldman, MD.)

become inflamed as a result of direct trauma or overuse of the joint. Other bursae susceptible to the development of bursitis exist between the insertion of the biceps and the head of the radius, as well as in the antecubital and cubital area.

CLINICAL SYNDROME

Tennis elbow (also known as lateral epicondylitis) is caused by repetitive microtrauma to the extensor tendons of the forearm. The pathophysiology of tennis elbow initially involves microtearing at the origin of the extensor carpi radialis and extensor carpi ulnaris. Secondary inflammation may become chronic as a result of continued overuse or misuse of the extensors of the forearm, and additional tendon damage may occur (Fig. 11.6). Coexistent bursitis, arthritis, or gout may perpetuate the pain and disability of tennis elbow.

The most common nidus of pain from tennis elbow is the bony origin of the extensor tendon of the extensor carpi radialis brevis at the anterior facet of the lateral epicondyle. Less commonly, tennis elbow pain originates from the origin of the extensor carpi radialis longus at the supracondylar crest; rarely, it originates more distally, at the point where the extensor carpi radialis brevis overlies the radial head. The olecranon bursa lies in the posterior aspect of the elbow joint and may also become inflamed (bursitis) as a result of direct trauma to the joint or its overuse. Other bursae susceptible to the development of bursitis lie between the insertion of the biceps and the head of the radius as well as in the antecubital and cubital areas. Tennis elbow occurs in individuals engaged in repetitive activities such as hand grasping (e.g., shaking hands) or high-torque wrist turning (e.g., scooping ice cream). Tennis players develop tennis elbow by two different mechanisms: (1) increased pressure grip strain as a result of playing with a too-heavy racket, and (2) making backhand shots with a leading shoulder and elbow rather than keeping the shoulder and elbow parallel to the net. Other racket sports players are also susceptible to the development of tennis elbow.

SIGNS AND SYMPTOMS

The pain of tennis elbow is localized to the region of the lateral epicondyle. This pain is constant and is made worse with active contraction of the wrist. Patients note the inability to hold a coffee cup or use a hammer. Sleep disturbance is common. On physical examination, tenderness is elicited along the extensor tendons at or just below the lateral epicondyle. Many patients with tennis elbow exhibit a bandlike thickening within the affected extensor tendons. Elbow range of motion is normal, but grip strength on the affected side is diminished. Patients with tennis elbow have a positive tennis elbow test result. This test is performed by stabilizing the patient's forearm and then having the patient clench the fist and actively extend the wrist. The examiner then attempts to force the wrist into flexion (see Fig. 11.2). Sudden, severe pain is highly suggestive of tennis elbow.

TESTING

Electromyography can help distinguish cervical radiculopathy and radial tunnel syndrome from tennis elbow. Plain radiographs should be obtained in all patients who present with elbow pain to rule out joint mice and other occult bony disease. Ultrasound imaging will help quantify the extent of tendinopathy and identify other occult causes of the patient's pain symptomatology (Fig. 11.7). Based on the patient's clinical presentation, additional testing may be warranted, including a complete blood count, uric acid level, erythrocyte sedimentation rate, and antinuclear antibody testing. Magnetic resonance imaging of the elbow is indicated if joint instability is suspected or if the symptoms of tennis elbow persist (see Fig. 11.4). The injection technique described later serves as both a diagnostic and a therapeutic maneuver.

DIFFERENTIAL DIAGNOSIS

Radial tunnel syndrome and, occasionally, C6–7 radiculopathy can mimic tennis elbow (Table 11.1). Radial tunnel syndrome is caused by entrapment of the radial nerve below the elbow. With radial tunnel syndrome, the maximal tenderness to palpation is distal to the lateral epicondyle over the radial nerve, whereas with tennis elbow, the maximal tenderness to palpation is over the lateral epicondyle (Fig. 11.8).

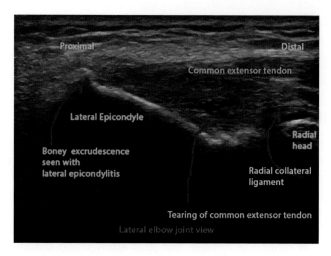

Fig. 11.7 As tennis elbow persists, bony abnormalities of the lateral epicondyle are commonly seen as demonstrated on this ultrasound image. (Courtesy Steven Waldman, MD.)

TABLE 11.1 ■ Characteristics of Radial Tunnel Syndrome and Lateral Epicondylitis

Characteristic	Radial Tunnel Syndrome	Lateral Epicondylitis (Tennis Elbow)
Frequency	Rare (2% of all peripheral nerve compressions of the upper limb)	Common cause of lateral elbow pain
Cause	Compression of the radial nerve	Caused by overuse of the extensor and supinator muscles
Characteristic patient	Anybody with repetitive, stressful pronation and supination (e.g., tennis players, Frisbee players, swimmers, powerlifters)	Tennis players
Pain location	Pain over the neck of the radius and lateral aspect of the proximal forearm over the extensor muscles themselves (distal to where the pain is located in lower extremity)	Pain and tenderness over the lateral epicondyle and immediately distal to it (at the origin of the extensor muscles)
Pain radiation	Pain can radiate proximally and (more commonly) distally	Usually localized without radiation
Provocative tests (much overlap between the two entities)	Pain with resisted extension of the middle finger with the forearm pronated and the elbow extended. Pain with resisted forearm supination with the elbow fully extended	Pain with resisted wrist extension or elbow supination with the elbow extended. Pain with forceful wrist flexion or forearm pronation

TREATMENT

Initial treatment of the pain and functional disability associated with tennis elbow includes a combination of nonsteroidal antiinflammatory drugs

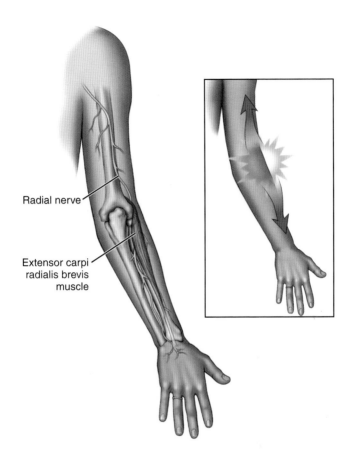

Radial nerve

Extensor carpi
radialis brevis
muscle

Fig. 11.8 The pain of radial tunnel syndrome is localized to the deep extensor muscle mass and may radiate proximally and distally into the upper arm and forearm. (From Waldman SD. *Atlas of Uncommon Pain Syndromes*. 3rd ed. Philadelphia, PA: Saunders; 2014 [Fig. 42.1].)

(NSAIDs) or cyclooxygenase-2 (COX-2) inhibitors and physical therapy. Local application of heat and cold may also be beneficial. Any repetitive activity that may exacerbate the patient's symptoms should be avoided. For patients who do not respond to these treatment modalities, injection of local anesthetic and steroid is a reasonable next step.

Injection for tennis elbow is performed by placing the patient in the supine position with the arm fully adducted at the patient's side, the elbow flexed, and the dorsum of the hand resting on a folded towel to relax the affected tendons. A total of 1 mL local anesthetic and 40 mg methylprednisolone is drawn up in a 5-mL sterile syringe. After sterile preparation of the skin overlying the posterolateral aspect of the joint, the lateral epicondyle is identified. Using strict aseptic technique, a 1-inch, 25-gauge needle is inserted perpendicular to the lateral

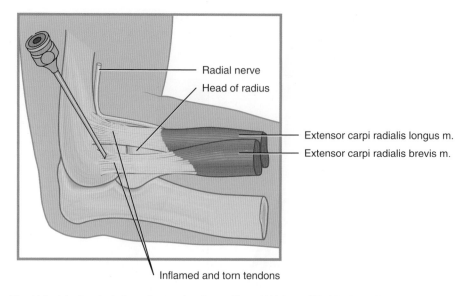

Fig. 11.9 Injection technique for tennis elbow. (From Waldman SD, Bloch J. *Pain Management*. Philadelphia: Saunders; 2007 [Fig. 63.5].)

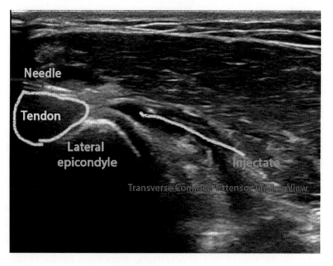

Fig. 11.10 Ultrasound-guided needle placement in a 31-year-old man with lateral epicondylitis. Ultrasound is well suited for needle tip visualization, allowing for precise placement for administration of platelet-rich plasma. (Courtesy Steven Waldman MD.)

epicondyle through the skin and into the subcutaneous tissue overlying the affected tendon (Fig. 11.9). If bone is encountered, the needle is withdrawn into the subcutaneous tissue. The contents of the syringe are then gently injected. Little resistance to injection should be felt. If resistance is encountered, the needle is probably in the tendon and should be withdrawn until the injection can proceed without significant resistance. The needle is then removed, and a sterile pressure dressing and ice pack are applied to the injection site. Recent clinical experience suggests that the injection of type A botulinum toxin and platelet-rich plasma and/or stem cells may provide improved symptom relief and healing of tennis elbow. Ultrasound guidance may improve the accuracy of needle placement in patients in whom anatomic landmarks are hard to identify (Fig. 11.10).

HIGH-YIELD TAKEAWAYS

- The patient is afebrile, making an acute infectious etiology (e.g., septic arthritis or bursitis) unlikely.
- The patient's symptomatology is thought to be the result of overuse from playing tennis with a heavy racquet.
- Physical examination and testing should be focused on the identification of infection and neurologic deficits.
- Radial tunnel syndrome should be considered in any patient thought to be suffering from tennis elbow.
- The patient has point tenderness over the lateral epicondyle.
- The patient's symptoms are unilateral and only involve one joint, which is more suggestive of a local process than a systemic polyarthropathy.
- The patient has a positive tennis elbow test.
- Plain radiographs will provide high-yield information regarding the bony contents of the joint, but ultrasound imaging and MRI will be more useful in identifying soft tissue pathology.
- Electromyography and nerve conduction velocity testing will help delineate the location and degree of nerve compromise, in particular ulnar nerve entrapment.

Suggested Readings

Waldman SD. Lateral epicondylitis injection. In: *Atlas of Pain Management Injection Techniques*. 4th ed. Philadelphia, PA: Elsevier; 2017:149–152.

Waldman SD. Radial tunnel syndrome. In: *Atlas of Uncommon Pain Syndromes*. 4th ed. Philadelphia, PA: Elsevier; 2019:113–117.

Waldman SD. Tennis elbow. In: *Atlas of Common Pain Syndromes*. 4th ed. Philadelphia, PA: Elsevier; 2019:149–152.

Waldman SD. Tennis elbow. In: *Pain Review*. 2nd ed. Philadelphia, PA: Saunders Elsevier; 2017:250–251.

Waldman SD. The tennis elbow test. In: *Physical Diagnosis of Pain. An Atlas of Signs and Symptoms*. 3rd ed. Philadelphia, PA: Elsevier; 2016:130–132.

CHAPTER
12

Nancy Givens

A 52-Year-Old Female With Medial Elbow Pain

Nancy Givens

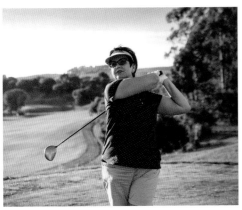

Nancy Givens is a 52-year-old book-keeper with the chief complaint of "right elbow pain." Nancy stated that over the past 5 or 6 weeks, she began noticing that her right elbow was becoming more and more pain-ful. Nancy stated that she was really worried about tax season because she was having a hard time using the mouse on her computer due to her elbow pain. I asked what she thought caused the elbow pain and she said, "I thought about that a lot, but really can't identify any specific event, although the pain first started when my friends and I went to Hilton Head for a golf weekend." She went on to say, "A couple of days, my squad played 27 holes." I asked what she had tried to make it better and she reported that Tylenol and the heating pad helped a little, but the pain came back whenever she grabbed her coffee mug, used the computer, or turned the doorknob to enter her condo. I asked Nancy if she had any numbness associated with her pain and she just shook her head but noted that she felt like her grip was weak. She denied any fever, chills, or other constitutional symptoms. Nancy denied significant sleep disturbance. I asked her about any antecedent elbow trauma and she just shook her head no.

I asked Nancy to point with one finger to show me where it hurt the most. She pointed to the medial epicondyle of the right elbow. "Doctor, it really hurts all around this area. I just don't know what is going on. Do you think I have arthritis?" I reassured her that together we would figure out what was going on and then we would get it better. "Just so it's in time for tax season, Doc."

On physical examination, Nancy was afebrile. Her respirations were 16 and her pulse was 72 and regular. Her blood pressure was 120/70. Nancy's head, eyes, ears, nose, throat (HEENT) exam was normal, as was her cardiopulmonary examination. Her thyroid was normal. Her abdominal examination revealed no abnormal mass or organomegaly. There was no costovertebral angle (CVA) tenderness. There was no peripheral edema. Her low back examination was unremarkable. Visual inspection of the right elbow revealed that the elbow was a little swollen medially. Palpation of the elbow revealed that the medial aspect was a little warm, but there was no obvious infection or olecranon bursitis. There was marked tenderness to pal-pation of the area overlying the right medial epicondyle of the elbow

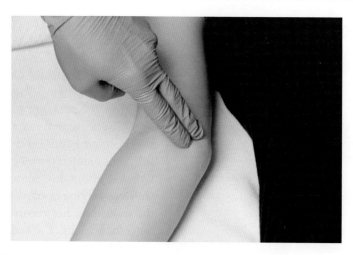

Fig. 12.1 Palpation of the medial epicondyle of the elbow will cause pain in patients suffering from golfer's elbow. (Courtesy Steven Waldman, MD.)

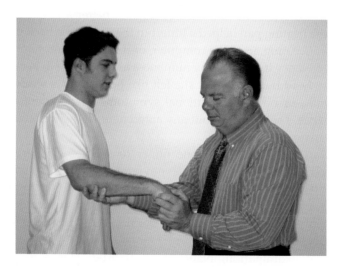

Fig. 12.2 The golfer's elbow test is performed by stabilizing the patient's forearm and then having the patient clench the fist and actively flex the wrist. The examiner then attempts to force the wrist into extension. Sudden, severe pain is highly suggestive of golfer's elbow. (From Waldman SD. *Physical Diagnosis of Pain*. 3rd ed. St Louis, MO: Elsevier; 2016 [Fig. 88.1].)

(Fig. 12.1). Nancy's golfer's elbow test was markedly positive on the right (Fig. 12.2). The left elbow examination was normal, as was examination of her other major joints. A careful neurologic examination of the upper extremities revealed that there was no evidence of peripheral neuropathy or entrapment neuropathy. Deep tendon reflexes were normal.

Key Clinical Points—What's Important and What's Not

THE HISTORY

- A history of onset of right medial elbow pain after a busy weekend of golf
- No history of previous significant elbow pain
- Weak grip strength
- No fever of chills
- Exacerbation of pain when lifting a coffee cup, using a computer mouse, and opening a door

THE PHYSICAL EXAMINATION

- The patient is afebrile
- Point tenderness to palpation of the area over the right medial epicondyle
- No evidence of entrapment neuropathy
- Warmth and slight swelling over the right medial epicondyle of the elbow
- Positive golfer's elbow test
- No evidence of infection

OTHER FINDINGS OF NOTE

- Normal HEENT examination
- Normal cardiovascular examination
- Normal pulmonary examination
- Normal abdominal examination
- No peripheral edema
- Normal upper extremity neurologic examination, motor and sensory examination
- Examination of other joints other than the right elbow were normal

 What Tests Would You Like to Order?

The following tests were ordered:
- Plain radiographs of the right elbow
- Ultrasound of the right elbow
- Magnetic resonance imaging (MRI) of the right elbow

TEST RESULTS

The plain radiographs of the right elbow revealed punctate calcifications within the common flexor tendon substance (Fig. 12.3A).

Ultrasound examination of the right elbow revealed tearing of the insertion of the common flexor tendon (see Fig. 12.3B—D).

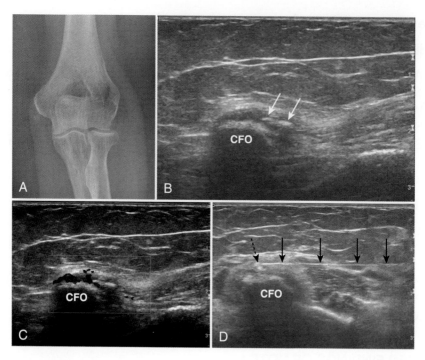

Fig. 12.3 (A) Radiograph of a middle-aged woman with golfer's elbow demonstrates a few small areas of calcification in the CFO adjacent to the medial epicondyle. (B, C) The corresponding ultrasound (US) images show an echo-poor tendon with small echogenic foci of calcification *(white arrows)* and neovascularization, as evident by increased blood flow on Doppler imaging (C) consistent with tendinopathy. (D) US-guided injection and dry needling shows the needle *(black arrows)* with the tip adjacent to the areas of calcification *(broken black arrow)*. *CFO,* Common flexor origin. (From Waldman SD. *Atlas of Common Pain Syndromes.* 4th ed. Philadelphia, PA: Elsevier; 2019 [Fig. 39.4].)

MRI scan of the right elbow revealed thickening and increased signal intensity of the common flexor tendon as well as bone marrow edema of the medial epicondyle (Fig. 12.4).

 ## Clinical Correlation—Putting It All Together

What is the diagnosis?
- Golfer's elbow (medial epicondylitis)

The Science Behind the Diagnosis
ANATOMY

The key landmarks when evaluating a patient for golfer's elbow are the flexor tendons of the pronator teres, flexor carpi radialis, flexor carpi

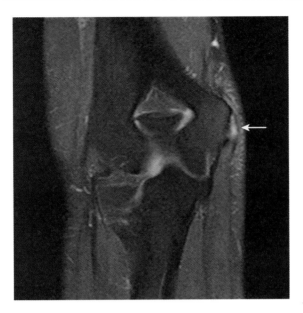

Fig. 12.4 T2-coronal magnetic resonance image of medial epicondylitis with a pathologic increase in signal intensity at the origin of the flexor-pronator mass *(arrow)*. (From Waldman SD. *Atlas of Common Pain Syndromes*. 4th ed. Philadelphia, PA: Elsevier; 2019 [Fig. 39.5].)

ulnaris, and palmaris muscles and their points of origin on the anterior facet of the medial epicondyle of the elbow (Figs. 12.5 and 12.6). Cubital and olecranon bursitis may coexist with golfer's elbow, further confusing the clinical presentations. The ulnar nerve is in proximity to the medial epicondyle and subject to needle-induced trauma during this injection technique. The nerve exits the axilla, and it passes inferiorly adjacent to the brachial artery. At the middle of the upper arm, the ulnar nerve turns medially to pass between the olecranon process and medial epicondyle of the humerus. Continuing its downward path, the ulnar nerve passes between the heads of the flexor carpi ulnaris, moving radially along with the ulnar artery.

CLINICAL SYNDROME

Although 15 times less common than tennis elbow, golfer's elbow remains one of the most common causes of elbow and forearm pain. Golfer's elbow (also known as medial epicondylitis) is caused by repetitive microtrauma to the flexor tendons of the forearm in a manner analogous to tennis elbow. The pathophysiology of golfer's elbow is initially caused by microtearing at the origins of the pronator teres, flexor carpi radialis, flexor carpi ulnaris, and the palmaris longus (Fig. 12.7). Secondary inflammation may occur that

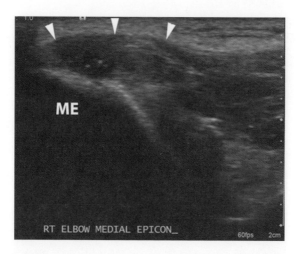

Fig. 12.5 Ultrasound image of golfer's elbow. *ME*, Medial epicondyle. Arrowheads indicate the common flexor tendon. Note the tendinosis and punctate calcifications within the tendon substance. (Courtesy Steven Waldman, MD.)

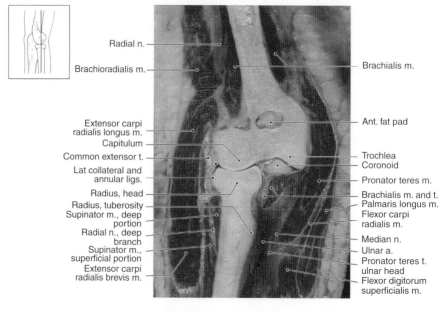

Fig. 12.6 Origins of the pronator teres, flexor carpi radialis, flexor carpi ulnaris, palmaris longus, and medial epicondyle. (From Waldman SD. *Atlas of Common Pain Syndromes*. 4th ed. Philadelphia, PA: Elsevier; 2019 [Fig. 39.1].)

can become chronic as the result of continued overuse or misuse of the flexors of the forearm. The most common nidus of pain from golfer's elbow is the bony origin of the flexor tendon of the flexor carpi radialis and the

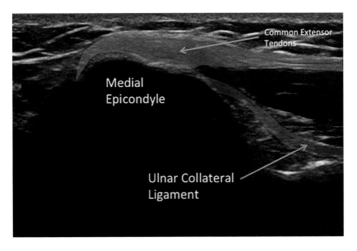

Fig. 12.7   Longitudinal ultrasound image of common flexor tendons. (Courtesy Steven Waldman, MD.)

humeral heads of the flexor carpi ulnaris and pronator teres at the medial epicondyle of the humerus (Fig. 12.8). Less commonly, golfer's elbow pain can originate from the ulnar head of the flexor carpi ulnaris at the medial aspect of the olecranon process. Coexisting bursitis, arthritis, and gout may also perpetuate the pain and disability of golfer's elbow. Golfer's elbow occurs in patients engaged in repetitive flexion activities that include throwing baseballs or footballs, carrying heavy suitcases, and driving golf balls (Fig. 12.9). These activities have in common repetitive flexion of the wrist and strain on the flexor tendons due to excessive weight or sudden arrested motion. Interestingly, many of the activities that can cause tennis elbow can also cause golfer's elbow.

SIGNS AND SYMPTOMS

The pain of golfer's elbow is localized to the region of the medial epicondyle (see Fig. 12.1). This pain is constant and is made worse with active contraction of the wrist. Patients note the inability to hold a coffee cup or use a hammer. Sleep disturbance is common. On physical examination, tenderness is elicited along the flexor tendons at or just below the medial epicondyle. Many patients with golfer's elbow exhibit a bandlike thickening within the affected flexor tendons. Elbow range of motion is normal, but grip strength on the affected side is diminished. Patients with golfer's elbow have a positive golfer's elbow test result. This test is performed by stabilizing the patient's forearm and then having the patient actively flex the wrist. The examiner then attempts to force the wrist into extension (see Fig. 12.2). Sudden, severe pain is highly suggestive of golfer's elbow.

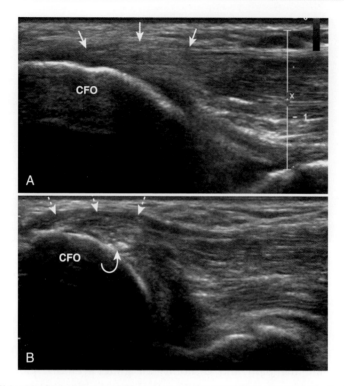

Fig. 12.8 (A) Longitudinal ultrasound (US) image of the asymptomatic elbow of a patient presenting with golfer's elbow. The common flexor origin *(CFO)* of the medial humeral epicondyle gives rise to a normal echogenic common flexor tendon *(white arrows)*. (B) On the affected side, the tendon is thickened with heterogeneous low-echo change *(broken white arrows)*, and there are small areas of echo-bright degenerative microcalcification *(curved white arrow)*. These US features are typical of insertional tendinopathy associated with golfer's or tennis elbow. (From Waldman SD, Campbell RSD. *Imaging of Pain*. Philadelphia, PA: Saunders; 2011 [Fig. 104.1].)

TESTING

Plain radiographs should be obtained in all patients who present with elbow pain to rule out joint mice and other occult bony disease. Based on the patient's clinical presentation, additional testing may be warranted, including a complete blood count, uric acid level, erythrocyte sedimentation rate, and antinuclear antibody testing. Ultrasound imaging will help quantify the extent of tendinopathy and identify other occult causes of the patient's pain symptomatology (see Fig. 12.5). Magnetic resonance imaging of the elbow is indicated if joint instability is suspected or if the symptoms of golfer's elbow persists (see Fig. 12.4). Electromyography (EMG) is indicated to diagnose entrapment neuropathy at the elbow and to distinguish golfer's elbow from cervical radiculopathy. The injection technique described later serves as both a diagnostic and a therapeutic maneuver.

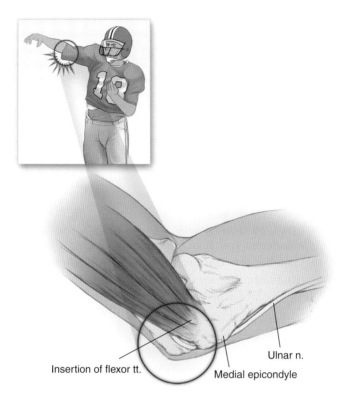

Fig. 12.9 The pain of golfer's elbow occurs at the medial epicondyle. (From Waldman SD. *Atlas of Common Pain Syndromes*. 4th ed. Philadelphia, PA: Elsevier; 2019 [Fig. 39.2].)

DIFFERENTIAL DIAGNOSIS

Occasionally, C6–7 radiculopathy mimics golfer's elbow; however, patients suffering from cervical radiculopathy usually have neck pain and proximal upper extremity pain in addition to symptoms below the elbow. As noted earlier, EMG can distinguish radiculopathy from golfer's elbow. Bursitis, arthritis, and gout may also mimic golfer's elbow, thus confusing the diagnosis. The olecranon bursa lies in the posterior aspect of the elbow joint and may become inflamed as a result of direct trauma to the joint or its overuse. Other bursae susceptible to the development of bursitis are located between the insertion of the biceps and the head of the radius, as well as in the antecubital and cubital areas.

TREATMENT

Initial treatment of the pain and functional disability associated with golfer's elbow includes a combination of nonsteroidal antiinflammatory drugs

(NSAIDs) or cyclooxygenase-2 (COX-2) inhibitors and physical therapy. Local application of heat and cold may also be beneficial. Any repetitive activity that may exacerbate the patient's symptoms should be avoided. For patients who do not respond to these treatment modalities, injection with local anesthetic and steroid is a reasonable next step.

Injection for golfer's elbow is carried out by placing the patient in the supine position with the arm fully adducted at the side, the elbow fully extended, and the dorsum of the hand resting on a folded towel to relax the affected tendons. A total of 1 mL local anesthetic and 40 mg methylprednisolone is drawn up in a 5-mL sterile syringe. After sterile preparation of the skin overlying the medial aspect of the joint, the medial epicondyle is identified. Using strict aseptic technique, a 1-inch, 25-gauge needle is inserted perpendicular to the medial epicondyle through the skin and into the subcutaneous tissue overlying the affected tendon. If bone is encountered, the needle is withdrawn into the subcutaneous tissue. The contents of the syringe are then gently injected. Little resistance to injection should be felt. If significant resistance is encountered, the needle is probably in the tendon and should be withdrawn until the injection can proceed with less resistance. The needle is then removed, and a sterile pressure dressing and ice pack are applied to the injection site. Recent clinical experience suggests that the injection of type A botulinum toxin and platelet-rich plasma and/or stem cells may provide improved symptom relief and healing of golfer's elbow. Ultrasound guidance may improve the accuracy of needle placement in patients in whom anatomic landmarks are hard to identify (Fig. 12.10).

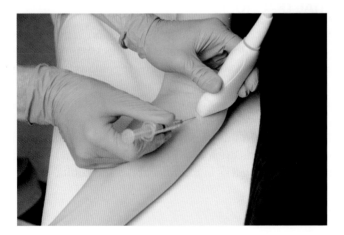

Fig. 12.10 Ultrasound-guided injection technique for golfer's elbow. (From Waldman SD. *Atlas of Common Pain Syndromes*. 4th ed. Philadelphia, PA: Elsevier; 2019 [Fig. 39.6].)

HIGH-YIELD TAKEAWAYS

- The patient is afebrile, making an acute infectious etiology (e.g., septic arthritis) unlikely.
- The patient's symptomatology is thought to be the result of overuse while playing golf.
- Physical examination and testing should be focused on the identification of infection and neurologic compromise.
- The patient has point tenderness over the medial epicondyle.
- The patient's symptoms are unimedial and only involve one joint, which is more suggestive of a local process than a systemic polyarthropathy.
- The patient has a positive golfer's elbow test.
- Plain radiographs will provide high-yield information regarding the bony contents of the joint, but ultrasound imaging and MRI will be more useful in identifying soft tissue pathology.
- Electromyography and nerve conduction velocity testing will help delineate the location and degree of nerve compromise.

Suggested Readings

McMurtrie A, Watts AC. Tennis elbow and golfer's elbow. *Orthop Trauma*. 2012;26 (5):337–344.

Pitzer ME, Seidenberg PH, Bader DA. Elbow tendinopathy. *Med Clin North Am*. 2014;98 (4):833–849.

Vinod AV, Ross G. An effective approach to diagnosis and surgical repair of refractory medial epicondylitis. *J Shoulder Elbow Surg*. 2015;24(8):1172–1177.

Waldman SD. Golfer's elbow. In: *Pain Review*. 2nd ed. Philadelphia, PA: Elsevier; 2017:251–252.

Waldman SD. Golfer's elbow and other abnormalities of the medial elbow. In: *Waldman's Comprehensive Atlas of Diagnostic Ultrasound of Painful Conditions*. Philadelphia: Wolters Kluwer; 2016:295–303.

Waldman SD. Medial epicondyle injection for golfer's elbow. In: *Atlas of Pain Management Injection Techniques*. 4th ed. Philadelphia: Elsevier; 2017:198–202.

Waldman SD, Campbell RSD. Golfer's elbow. In: *Imaging of Pain*. Philadelphia: Saunders; 2011:263–264.

Alan Winnie

A 62-Year-Old Male With Posterior Elbow Pain and Swelling

- Learn the common causes of elbow pain.
- Develop an understanding of the unique anatomy of the elbow joint.
- Develop an understanding of the anatomy of the olecranon bursa.
- Develop an understanding of the bursae of the elbow.
- Develop an understanding of the causes of olecranon bursitis.
- Develop an understanding of the differential diagnosis of olecranon bursitis.
- Learn the clinical presentation of olecranon bursitis.
- Learn how to examine the elbow.
- Learn how to use physical examination to identify olecranon bursitis.
- Develop an understanding of the treatment options for olecranon bursitis.

Alan Winnie

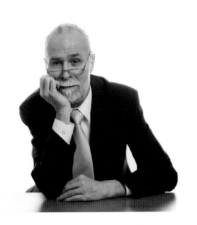

Alan Winnie is a 62-year-old architect with the chief complaint of "My right elbow is so swollen that I can't put on my dress shirt." Alan stated that over the past few weeks he began noticing that his right elbow was becoming more and more swollen and painful. Alan stated that he was really worried that he "might have cancer, the way my elbow had swollen up." I reassured Alan that we would get it sorted out and that we would get him the answers that he needed. I asked Alan what he thought caused the elbow swelling and pain, and he said that he had "been burning the midnight oil trying to complete plans for the airport and had been doing a lot of drawing." He noted that by the end of the day, his right elbow was getting sore. He tried putting a towel under the elbow to pad it, but it really didn't help the pain. He noted that the back of his elbow began to "feel squishy" and over the last week, it had "swollen up to three times its normal size." I asked what he had tried to make it better and he said that he felt like the heating pad made it worse and that the pain pills he borrowed from his partner did nothing but make him feel sick to his stomach. "I tried an Ace wrap, but all it did was make my elbow hurt even more." I asked Alan if he had any numbness associated with his pain and he just shook his head, but again expressed concern that this was the "Big C." After again reassuring him, I asked Alan about any fever, chills, or other constitutional symptoms such as weight loss, night sweats, etc. and he just shook his head no. He denied any antecedent elbow trauma, but noted that sometimes the elbow pain woke him up at night.

I asked Alan to point with one finger to show me where it hurt the most. He pointed to the right olecranon process, where I noted a massive accumulation of fluid (Fig. 13.1). I told Alan I thought I had a pretty good idea that it was not cancer and reassured him that together, we would figure out what was going on and then we would get it better. He replied, "From your mouth to God's ears, Doc."

On physical examination, Alan was afebrile. His respirations were 16, his pulse was 72 and regular, and his blood pressure was 120/70. Alan's head, eyes, ears, nose, throat (HEENT) exam was normal, as was his cardiopulmonary examination. His thyroid was normal. His abdominal examination revealed no abnormal mass or organomegaly. There was no costovertebral angle (CVA) tenderness. There was no peripheral edema. His low back examination was unremarkable. Visual inspection of the right elbow revealed that there was a large

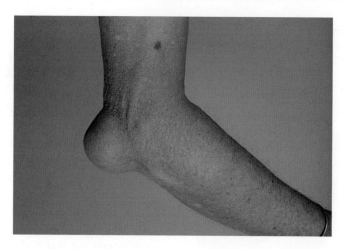

Fig. 13.1 Classic olecranon bursitis. (From Waldman SD, Bloch J. *Pain Management*. Philadelphia, PA: Saunders; 2007 [Fig. 65.1].)

accumulation of fluid overlying the olecranon process. The posterior elbow was warm to touch, there was slight rubor, and the swollen area was not fluctuant. There was no obvious infection. There was marked tenderness to palpation of the area overlying the olecranon process (see Fig. 13.1). Passive and active flexion and extension of Alan's elbow reproduced his pain. The left elbow examination was normal, as was examination of his other major joints. Specifically, there was no evidence of rheumatoid or other inflammatory arthritis. A careful neurologic examination of the upper extremities revealed that there was no evidence of peripheral neuropathy or entrapment neuropathy of the ulnar nerves. Deep tendon reflexes were normal.

Key Clinical Points—What's Important and What's Not
THE HISTORY

- A history of the onset of right posterior elbow pain and swelling associated with prolonged and repeated resting of the affected elbow on a desk
- No history of previous significant elbow pain or swelling
- No fever of chills
- Concern that the significant swelling might be cancer

THE PHYSICAL EXAMINATION

- The patient is afebrile
- Massive swelling over the posterior elbow
- Tenderness to palpation of the area over the right olecranon process

- No evidence of entrapment neuropathy of the ulnar nerve
- Warmth over the posterior elbow
- Slight rubor of the posterior elbow
- No evidence of infection
- No evidence of rheumatoid or other inflammatory arthritis

OTHER FINDINGS OF NOTE

- Normal HEENT examination
- Normal cardiovascular examination
- Normal pulmonary examination
- Normal abdominal examination
- No peripheral edema
- Normal upper extremity neurologic examination, motor and sensory examination
- Examination of other joints other than the right elbow were normal

 ## What Tests Would You Like to Order?

The following tests were ordered:
- Plain radiographs of the right elbow
- Ultrasound of the right elbow
- Magnetic resonance imaging (MRI) of the right elbow

TEST RESULTS

The plain radiographs of the right elbow revealed significant soft tissue swelling consistent with olecranon bursitis (Fig. 13.2).

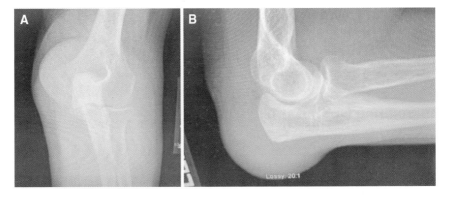

Fig. 13.2 (A) Anteroposterior and (B) lateral radiographs of a patient with olecranon bursitis. (From Reilly D, Kamineni S. Olecranon bursitis. *J Shoulder Elbow Surg*. 2016;25(1):158–167 [Fig. 9].)

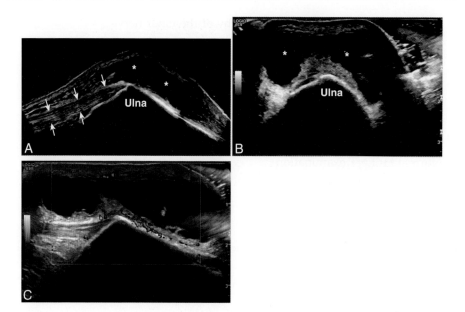

Fig. 13.3 Longitudinal (A) and axial (B) ultrasound (US) images of a patient with olecranon bursitis. There is a low-echo, fluid-filled bursa *(asterisks)* superficial to the proximal ulna, and the distal triceps tendon is visualized on the longitudinal image *(white arrows)*. (C) The Doppler US image demonstrates increased vascularity in the periphery of the bursa, consistent with mild inflammatory synovitis. (From Waldman SD, Campbell RSD. *Imaging of Pain*. Philadelphia, PA: Saunders; 2011 [Fig. 108.1].)

Ultrasound examination of the right elbow revealed a fluid-filled bursa (Fig. 13.3).

MRI scan of the right elbow revealed thickening and increased signal intensity of the common flexor tendon as well as bone marrow edema of the medial epicondyle (Fig. 13.4).

Clinical Correlation—Putting It All Together

What is the diagnosis?
- Olecranon bursitis (medial epicondylitis)

The Science Behind the Diagnosis
ANATOMY

The elbow joint is a synovial, hinge-type joint that serves as the articulation between the humerus, radius, and ulna. The joint's primary function is to position the wrist to optimize hand function. The joint allows flexion and extension at the elbow, as well as pronation and supination of the forearm.

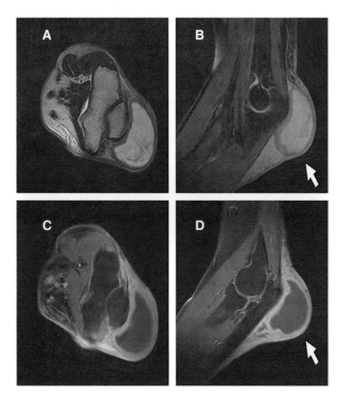

Fig. 13.4 Case 1: (A) axial T2-weighted fast spin echo magnetic resonance (MR) image showing distended olecranon bursa with thickened walls. (B) Sagittal T2 FAT SAT showing the same features with subcutaneous edema, (C) axial, (D) sagittal T1 FAT SAT post contrast showing enhancing margins with fluid distension and peribursal subcutaneous inflammation. (From Emad Y, Ragab Y, El-Shaarawy N, et al. Olecranon bursitis as initial presentation of gout in asymptomatic normouricemic patients. *Egypt Rheumatol.* 2014;36(1):47−50 [Fig. 2].)

The joint is lined with synovium. The entire joint is covered by a dense capsule that thickens medially to form the ulnar collateral ligament and laterally to form the radial collateral ligaments (Fig. 13.5A). These dense ligaments, coupled with the elbow joint's deep bony socket, make this joint extremely stable and relatively resistant to subluxation and dislocation. The anterior and posterior joint capsule is less dense and may become distended if there is a joint effusion. The olecranon bursa lies in the posterior aspect of the elbow joint between the olecranon process of the ulna and the overlying skin (see Fig. 13.5B). The olecranon bursa may become inflamed as a result of direct trauma or overuse of the joint. The elbow joint is innervated primarily by the musculocutaneous and radial nerves, with the ulnar and median nerves providing varying degrees of innervation. At the middle of the upper arm, the ulnar nerve courses medially to pass between the olecranon process and medial epicondyle of the humerus. The nerve is susceptible to

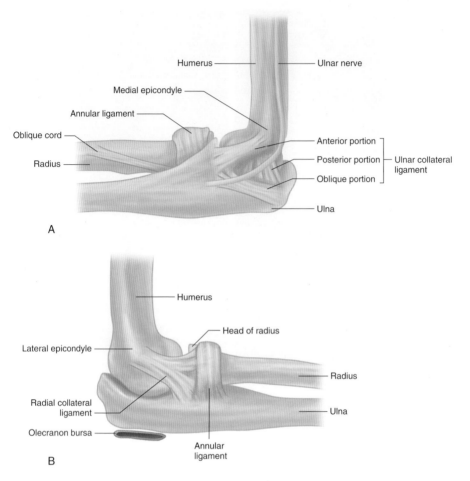

Fig. 13.5 (A) Ligaments of the posterior elbow and the relationship of the ulnar nerve to the olecranon process. (B) The olecranon bursa. (From Fam A, Lawry G, Kreder H. *Musculoskeletal Examination and Joint Injection Techniques*. Philadelphia, PA: Mosby; 2006 [Fig. 4.2].)

entrapment and trauma at this point. At the elbow, the median nerve lies just medial to the brachial artery and occasionally is damaged during brachial artery cannulation for blood gases.

CLINICAL SYNDROME

Olecranon bursitis may develop gradually as a result of repetitive irritation of the olecranon bursa or acutely as a result of trauma or infection. The olecranon bursa lies in the posterior aspect of the elbow between the olecranon process of the ulna and the overlying skin (see Fig. 13.5B). It may exist as a single bursal sac or, in some patients, a multisegmented series of loculated

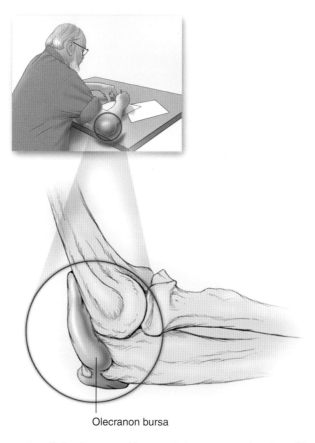

Olecranon bursa

Fig. 13.6   Olecranon bursitis is often caused by repeated pressure on the elbow. (From Waldman SD. *Atlas of Common Pain Syndromes*. 4th ed. Philadelphia, PA: Elsevier; 2019 [Fig. 48.1].)

sacs. With overuse or misuse, these bursae may become inflamed, enlarged, and on rare occasions, infected. The swelling associated with olecranon bursitis may be quite impressive, and the patient may complain about being unable to wear a long-sleeved shirt.

The olecranon bursa is vulnerable to injury from both acute trauma and repeated microtrauma. Acute injuries are often caused by direct trauma to the elbow in patients who play sports, such as hockey, or who fall directly onto the olecranon process. Repeated pressure from leaning on the elbow, such as when working long hours at a drafting table, may result in inflammation and swelling of the olecranon bursa (Fig. 13.6). Rarely, gout or bacterial infection precipitates acute olecranon bursitis. If inflammation of the olecranon bursa becomes chronic, rice bodies may occur, as may cords, as well as calcification of the bursa, resulting in residual calcified nodules called gravel (Fig. 13.7).

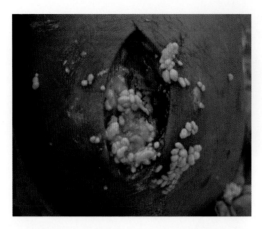

Fig. 13.7 Intraoperative photograph of a patient with rheumatoid arthritis and chronic olecranon bursitis. Abundant rice bodies were found when the bursa was excised. (From Waldman SD. *Atlas of Common Pain Syndromes*. 4th ed. Philadelphia, PA: Elsevier; 2019 [Fig. 48.2].)

BOX 13.1 ■ Other Names for Olecranon Bursitis

Draftsman's elbow
Plumber's elbow
Student's elbow
Miner's elbow
Dialysis elbow
Old man's bursitis

SIGNS AND SYMPTOMS

Patients suffering from olecranon bursitis, which is also known as dialysis elbow (among other descriptive names), frequently complain of swelling and pain with any movement of the elbow, but especially with extension (Box 13.1). The pain is localized to the olecranon area, with referred pain often noted above the elbow joint. Frequently, the patient is more concerned about the swelling than about the pain. Physical examination reveals point tenderness over the olecranon and swelling of the bursa that may be extensive (Fig. 13.8). Passive extension and resisted flexion reproduce the pain, as does any pressure over the bursa. Fever and chills usually accompany infection of the bursa.

TESTING

The diagnosis of olecranon bursitis is usually made on clinical grounds alone. Plain radiographs of the posterior elbow are indicated if the patient has a history

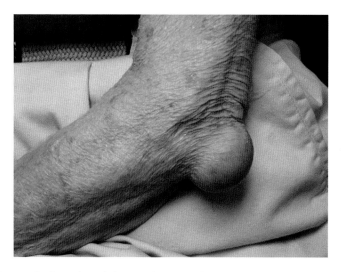

Fig. 13.8   Photograph of an enlarged olecranon bursa consistent with nonseptic olecranon bursitis. (From Waldman SD. *Atlas of Common Pain Syndromes*. 4th ed. Philadelphia, PA: Elsevier; 2019 [Fig. 48.3].)

of elbow trauma or if arthritis of the elbow is suspected. Plain radiographs may also reveal calcification of the bursa and associated structures consistent with chronic inflammation (see Fig. 13.2). If joint instability is suspected, magnetic resonance imaging and ultrasound imaging are indicated to further characterize the nature of masses of the posterior elbow (e.g., solid or cystic) and to clarify the diagnosis of olecranon bursitis if it is in question (see Figs. 13.3 and 13.4). A complete blood count, automated chemistry profile including uric acid level, erythrocyte sedimentation rate, and antinuclear antibody testing should be performed if collagen vascular disease is suspected. If infection is suspected, aspiration, Gram stain, and culture of the bursal fluid, followed by treatment with appropriate antibiotics, are required on an emergency basis.

DIFFERENTIAL DIAGNOSIS

Olecranon bursitis is usually a straightforward clinical diagnosis. Occasionally, rheumatoid nodules or gouty arthritis of the elbow may confuse the clinical picture. Synovial cysts of the elbow may also mimic olecranon bursitis. Coexistent tendinitis (e.g., tennis elbow, golfer's elbow) may require additional treatment. Rarely, pyoderma gangrenosa may mimic the clinical presentation of olecranon bursitis.

TREATMENT

A short course of conservative therapy consisting of simple analgesics, nonsteroidal antiinflammatory drugs (NSAIDs), or cyclooxygenase-2 (COX-2)

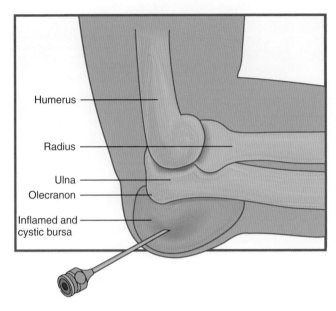

Fig. 13.9 Injection of the olecranon bursa. (From Waldman SD. *Atlas of Pain Management Injection Techniques*. 4th ed. St Louis, MO: Elsevier; 2017 [Fig. 58.4].)

inhibitors, along with an elbow protector to prevent further trauma, is the initial treatment for patients suffering from olecranon bursitis. If rapid improvement fails to occur, the following injection technique is a reasonable next step (Fig. 13.9). The patient is placed in the supine position with the arm fully adducted at the side, the elbow flexed, and the palm of the hand resting on the patient's abdomen. A total of 2 mL local anesthetic and 40 mg methylprednisolone is drawn up in a 5-mL sterile syringe. After sterile preparation of the skin overlying the posterior aspect of the joint, the olecranon process and overlying bursa are identified. Using strict aseptic technique, the clinician inserts a 1-inch, 25-gauge needle through the skin and subcutaneous tissues directly into the bursa in the midline. If bone is encountered, the needle is withdrawn into the bursa. The contents of the syringe are gently injected; little resistance to injection should be felt. The needle is removed, and a sterile pressure dressing and ice pack are applied to the injection site. Ultrasound needle guidance may be useful when draining a complex loculated or multisegmented olecranon bursa. Physical modalities, including local heat and gentle range of motion exercises, should be introduced several days after injection for elbow pain (Fig. 13.10). A compression dressing may also help prevent the reaccumulation of fluid following aspiration. Rarely, surgical removal of the inflamed bursa is required to relieve the pain and functional disability. Vigorous exercises should be avoided because they will exacerbate the patient's symptoms.

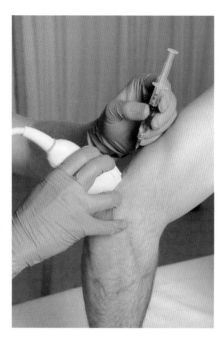

Fig. 13.10   Ultrasound-guided injection of the olecranon bursa. (Courtesy Steven Waldman, MD.)

HIGH-YIELD TAKEAWAYS

- The patient is afebrile, making an acute infectious etiology (e.g., septic bursitis) unlikely.
- The patient's symptomatology is thought to be the result of prolonged pressure on the right olecranon bursa.
- Physical examination and testing should be focused on the identification of infection or inflammatory causes of the olecranon bursitis.
- The patient exhibits massive swelling of the posterior elbow that is the classic presentation of olecranon bursitis.
- The patient's symptoms are unilateral and only involve one joint, which is more suggestive of a local process than a systemic inflammatory process.
- Plain radiographs will provide high-yield information regarding the bony contents of the joint, but ultrasound imaging and MRI will be more useful in identifying soft tissue pathology.
- Electromyography and nerve conduction velocity testing will help delineate the location and degree of nerve compromise if ulnar nerve compromise is suspected.

Suggested Readings

Reilly D, Kamineni S. Olecranon bursitis. *J Shoulder Elbow Surg*. 2016;25(1):158−167.

Waldman SD. Olecranon bursa injection. In: *Atlas of Pain Management Injection Techniques*. 4th ed. Philadelphia, PA: Elsevier; 2017:207−210.

Waldman SD. Olecranon bursitis. In: *Pain Review*. 2nd ed. Philadelphia, PA: Elsevier; 2017:257−258.

Waldman SD. Olecranon bursitis. In: *Waldman's Comprehensive Atlas of Diagnostic Ultrasound of Painful Conditions*. Philadelphia, PA: Wolters Kluwer; 2016:269−275.

Waldman SD, Campbell RSD. Olecranon bursitis. In: *Imaging of Pain*. Philadelphia, PA: Saunders; 2011:273−274.

Working S, Tyser A, Levy D. Mycobacterium avium complex olecranon bursitis resolves without antimicrobials or surgical intervention: a case report and review of the literature. *ID Cases*. 2015;2(2):59−62.

Yari SS, Reichel LM. Case report: misdiagnosed olecranon bursitis: pyoderma gangrenosum. *J Shoulder Elbow Surg*. 2014;23(9):e207−e211.

Johan Ryan

A 32-Year-Old Male With Pain and Electric Shocklike Sensation Radiating Into the Lateral Forearm and Ring and Little Finger

- Learn the common causes of forearm pain.
- Learn the common causes of hand numbness.
- Develop an understanding of the unique relationship of the ulnar nerve to the bones of the elbow.
- Develop an understanding of the anatomy of the ulnar nerve.
- Develop an understanding of the bursae of the elbow.
- Develop an understanding of the causes of tardy ulnar palsy.
- Develop an understanding of the differential diagnosis of tardy ulnar palsy.
- Learn the clinical presentation of tardy ulnar palsy.
- Learn how to examine the elbow.
- Learn how to examine the ulnar nerve.
- Learn how to use physical examination to identify tardy ulnar palsy.
- Develop an understanding of the treatment options for tardy ulnar palsy.

Johan Ryan

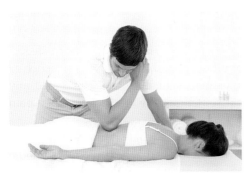

Johan Ryan is a 32-year-old massage therapist with the chief complaint of "pain and numbness in the side of my forearm and electric shocks into my ring finger and little finger." Johan stated that over the past several months, he began noticing a deep, aching sensation in his lateral forearm. It was associated with electric shocklike pains into the ring finger and little finger on the right. I asked Johan if he had experienced any numbness or weakness and he replied, "Doc, it's funny that you asked, as I am having the hardest time getting my keys out of my pants pocket because my little finger keeps catching on the edge of the pocket. And after a day at work, I have begun to notice that my little finger and part of my right ring finger—the part next to my little finger—are numb!" (Fig. 14.1). I asked Johan what he thought was causing his symptoms and he said that he wondered if it was related to using his elbow to massage his clients' spines. He said, "To do it correctly, it's bone against bone." I asked what he had tried to make it better and he said that

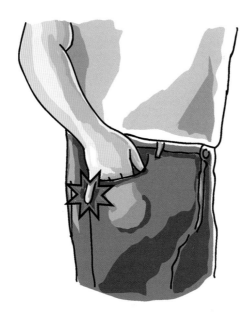

Fig. 14.1 The Wartenberg sign test for the ulnar nerve entrapment at the elbow. (From Waldman S: *Physical Diagnosis of Pain: An Atlas of Signs and Symptoms.* 3rd ed. St Louis, MO: Elsevier; 2016 [Fig. 78.2].)

he used a heating pad at night and it "seemed to make the pain better, but the numbness in my fingers is worse. Tylenol PM seemed to help some, at least with sleep." I asked Johan to describe any numbness he noticed associated with his pain and he pointed to his right little and ulnar aspect of his ring finger. "Doc, the whole little finger is numb, but just part of my ring finger goes to sleep." I asked Johan about any fever, chills, or other constitutional symptoms such as weight loss, night sweats, etc., and he just shook his head no. He denied any antecedent elbow trauma but noted that sometimes the electric shocklike pain woke him up at night.

I asked Johan to point with one finger to show me where it hurt the most. He pointed to the right lateral forearm. He went on to say that he could live with the pain, but the electric shocks and numbness were really bothering him. He then asked, "Doc, could this have anything to do with my rheumatoid arthritis?"

On physical examination, Johan was afebrile. His respirations were 18, his pulse was 74 and regular, and his blood pressure was 110/68. His HEENT (head, eyes, ears, nose, throat) exam was normal, as was his cardiopulmonary examination. His thyroid was normal. His abdominal examination revealed no abnormal mass or organomegaly. There was no CVA tenderness. There was no peripheral edema. His low back examination was unremarkable. Visual inspection of the right elbow was unremarkable. There was no rubor or color. There was no obvious infection or olecranon bursitis. There was a positive Tinel sign over the ulnar nerve at the elbow (Fig. 14.2). Repetitive active flexion and extension of Johan's elbow elicited paresthesias into the little finger and ulnar aspect of the ring finger on the right. Examination of Johan's hands revealed mild synovitis and mild ulnar drift consistent with his diagnosis of rheumatoid arthritis. The left elbow examination was normal, but there was mild crepitus on passive flexion and extension of his right elbow. A careful neurologic examination of the upper extremities revealed decreased sensation in the distribution of the ulnar nerve, as well as weakness of the intrinsic muscles of the right hand and weakness to the adductor pollicis brevis and flexor pollicis brevis (Fig. 14.3). Deep tendon reflexes were normal. Johan exhibited a positive Froment sign as well as a little finger adduction sign (Figs. 14.4 and 14.5). Jeanne sign was also positive (Fig. 14.6).

Key Clinical Points—What's Important and What's Not
THE HISTORY

- A history of the onset of right lateral forearm pain with associated paresthesias into the distribution of the ulnar nerve
- Numbness of the little finger and ulnar aspect of the ring finger on the right
- Hand weakness
- No history of previous significant elbow pain

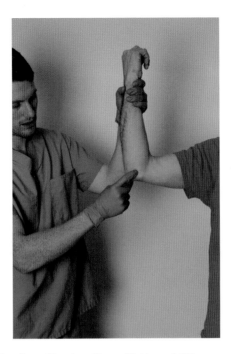

Fig. 14.2 Tinel's test at the elbow. (Courtesy Steven Waldman, MD.)

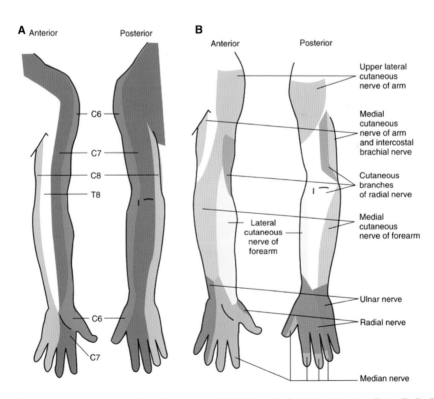

Fig. 14.3 Distribution of the ulnar nerve. (A) Dermatomos. (B) Peripheral nerves. (From Duffy BJ, Tubog TD. The prevention and recognition of ulnar nerve and brachial plexus injuries. *J PeriAnesth Nurs.* 2017;32(6):636−649 [Fig. 3].)

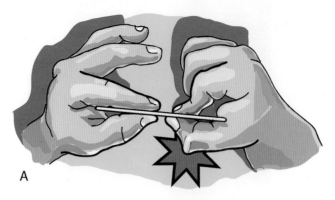

Fig. 14.4 Froment's sign is elicited by asking the patient to grasp a piece of paper lightly between the thumb and index finger of each hand and monitoring flexion of the thumb interphalangeal joint on the affected side. (From Waldman SD. *Atlas of Common Pain Syndromes*. 4th ed. Philadelphia, PA: Elsevier; 2019 [Fig. 45.2A].)

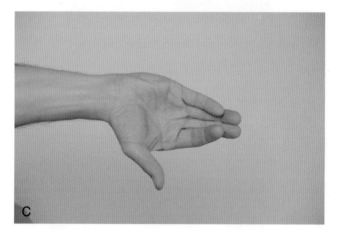

Fig. 14.5 The little finger adduction test evaluates the strength in the interosseous muscles of the hand that are innervated by the ulnar nerve. It is performed by asking the patient to touch the little finger to the index finger. (From Waldman SD. *Atlas of Common Pain Syndromes*. 4th ed. Philadelphia: Elsevier; 2019 [Fig. 45.2C].)

- Past medical history of rheumatoid arthritis
- No fever of chills

THE PHYSICAL EXAMINATION

- The patient is afebrile
- Positive Tinel sign at the elbow (see Fig. 14.2)
- Positive Wartenberg, Jeanne, Froment, and little finger adduction tests (see Figs. 14.1, 14.4, 14.5, and 14.6)

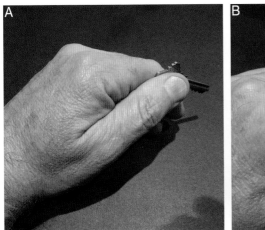
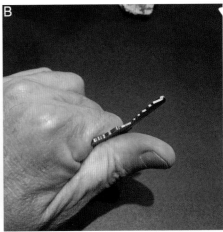

Fig. 14.6 (A) The Jeanne test is performed by asking the patient to lightly grasp a key between the thumb and radial aspect of the index finger of each hand and monitoring the flexion of the thumb interphalangeal joint on the affected side. (B) The patient is then asked to grasp the key more tightly. The Jeanne test is positive if the metacarpophalangeal joint of the affected thumb hyperextends to stabilize the joint to increase grasp pressure. (Courtesy Steven Waldman, MD.)

- Weakness of the intrinsic muscles of the right hand
- Numbness of the little and ring fingers in the distribution of the ulnar nerve (see Fig. 14.3)
- Hand findings suggestive of rheumatoid arthritis, including mild synovitis and ulnar drift
- No evidence of infection

OTHER FINDINGS OF NOTE

- Normal HEENT examination
- Normal cardiovascular examination
- Normal pulmonary examination
- Normal abdominal examination
- No peripheral edema
- Normal left upper extremity neurologic examination, motor and sensory examination

 What Tests Would You Like to Order?

The following tests were ordered:
- Plain radiographs of the right elbow
- Ultrasound of the right elbow
- Magnetic resonance imaging (MRI) of the right elbow

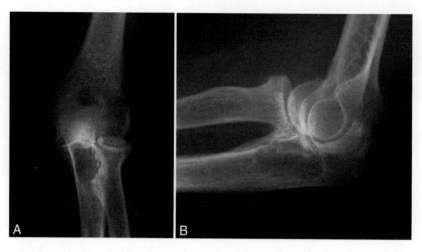

Fig. 14.7 Anteroposterior (AP) (A) and lateral (B) radiographs of early rheumatoid involvement of the elbow. There is global joint space narrowing, and a large lucent geode is present within the proximal ulna. No erosions are present. (From Waldman SD, Campbell RSD. *Imaging of Pain*. Philadelphia, PA: Saunders; 2011 [Fig. 110.1].)

- Electromyography (EMG) and nerve conduction velocity testing of the right upper extremity

TEST RESULTS

The plain radiographs of the right elbow revealed joint narrowing consistent with early rheumatoid involvement of the elbow (Fig. 14.7).

Ultrasound examination of the right elbow revealed compression of the ulnar nerve by synovitis secondary to rheumatoid arthritis (Fig. 14.8).

MRI scan of the right elbow reveals fibrous synovial pannus and joint effusion (Fig. 14.9).

EMG and nerve conduction velocity testing revealed slowing of ulnar nerve conduction across the elbow as well as denervation of the intrinsic muscles of the hand.

 Clinical Correlation—Putting It All Together

What is the diagnosis?
- Tardy ulnar palsy

The Science Behind the Diagnosis
ANATOMY

The ulnar nerve is made up of fibers from C6-T1 spinal roots. The nerve lies anterior and inferior to the axillary artery in the 3-o'clock–to–6-o'clock quadrant.

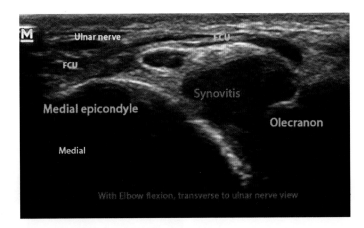

Fig. 14.8 Transverse ultrasound image of the elbow in the flexed position demonstrating compression of the ulnar nerve by exuberant synovitis in a patient suffering from rheumatoid arthritis. *FCU,* Flexor carpi ulnaris. (Courtesy Steven Waldman, MD.)

Exiting the axilla, the ulnar nerve descends into the upper arm along with the brachial artery. At the middle of the upper arm, the nerve courses medially to pass between the olecranon process and medial epicondyle of the humerus (Fig. 14.10). The nerve then passes between the heads of the flexor carpi ulnaris muscle continuing downward, moving radially along with the ulnar artery. At a point approximately 1 inch proximal to the crease of the wrist, the ulnar nerve divides into the dorsal and palmar branches. The dorsal branch provides sensation to the ulnar aspect of the dorsum of the hand and the dorsal aspect of the little finger and the ulnar half of the ring finger. The palmar branch provides sensory innervation to the ulnar aspect of the palm of the hand and the palmar aspect of the little finger and the ulnar half of the ring finger.

CLINICAL SYNDROME

Ulnar nerve entrapment at the elbow is one of the most common entrapment neuropathies encountered in clinical practice. The causes include compression of the ulnar nerve by an aponeurotic band that runs from the medial epicondyle of the humerus to the medial border of the olecranon, direct trauma to the ulnar nerve at the elbow, and repetitive elbow motion (see Fig. 14.10). Ulnar nerve entrapment at the elbow is also called tardy ulnar palsy, cubital tunnel syndrome, and ulnar nerve neuritis. This entrapment neuropathy manifests as pain and associated paresthesias in the lateral forearm, which radiate to the wrist and ring and little finger. Some patients suffering from ulnar nerve entrapment at the elbow may also notice pain referred to the medial aspect of the scapula on the affected side. Untreated,

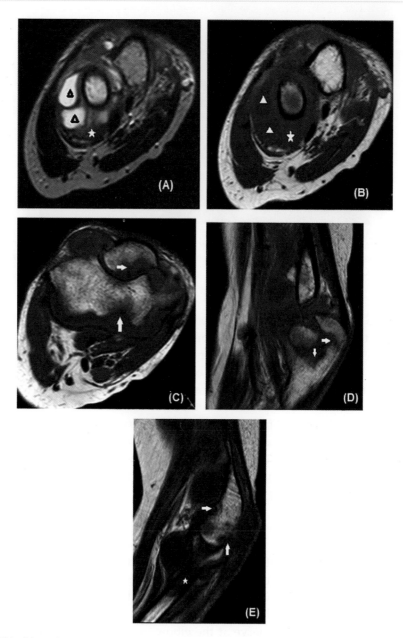

Fig. 14.9 Magnetic resonance imaging (MRI) of the elbow. (A) Axial T2-weighted and (B) T1-weighted MR images through the level of the proximal radioulnar joint reveal distension of the joint capsule with underlying low to intermediate signal fibrous synovial pannus *(asterisks)* and joint effusion *(triangles)*. (C) Axial and (D) sagittal T1-weighted MRI through the level of the ulnohumeral joint shows location and degree of marginal erosive changes *(arrows)*. (E) Sagittal T1-weighted MRI through level of the radiocapitellar joint reveals the anterior and posterior capitellar erosion and proximal radial bone marrow edema *(asterisk)*. (From Hasan NHA, Alam-Eldean MH, Mousa SS. Stiff elbow in adult: MR imaging findings. *Egypt J Radiol Nuclear Med*. 2015;46(4):1037−1048 [Fig. 6].)

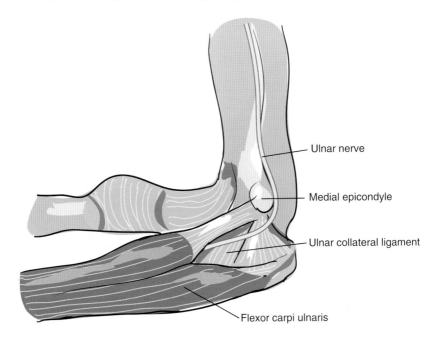

Fig. 14.10 The causes of ulnar nerve entrapment at the elbow include compression of the ulnar nerve by an aponeurotic band that runs from the medial epicondyle of the humerus to the medial border of the olecranon, direct trauma to the ulnar nerve at the elbow, and repetitive elbow motion. (From Waldman S, Bloch J. *Pain Management*. Philadelphia, PA: Saunders; 2007 [Fig. 66.1].)

ulnar nerve entrapment at the elbow can result in a progressive motor deficit, and ultimately flexion contracture of the affected fingers can result. The onset of symptoms is usually after repetitive elbow motion or from repeated pressure on the elbow, such as using the elbows to arise from bed. Direct trauma to the ulnar nerve as it enters the cubital tunnel may also result in a similar clinical presentation. Patients with vulnerable nerve syndrome (e.g., diabetics, alcoholics) are at greater risk for the development of ulnar nerve entrapment at the elbow (Fig. 14.11).

SIGNS AND SYMPTOMS

Physical findings include tenderness over the ulnar nerve at the elbow. A positive Tinel sign over the ulnar nerve as it passes beneath the aponeuroses is usually present. Weakness of the intrinsic muscles of the forearm and hand that are innervated by the ulnar nerve may be identified with careful manual muscle testing, although early in the course of the evolution of cubital tunnel syndrome, the only physical finding other than tenderness over the nerve may be the loss of sensation on the ulnar side of the little finger. Muscle wasting of the intrinsic muscles of the hand can best be identified by viewing the hand with the palm

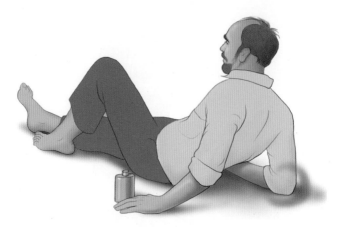

Fig. 14.11 The ulnar nerve is susceptible to compression at the elbow. (From Waldman SD, Bloch J. *Pain Management*. Philadelphia, PA: Saunders; 2007 [Fig. 66.3].)

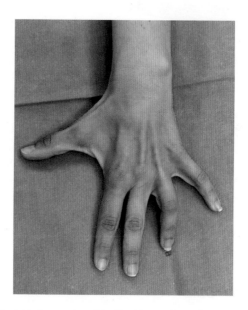

Fig. 14.12 Wasting of the intrinsic muscles of the hand in a patient with sever ulnar nerve entrapment at the elbow. (From Lauretti L, D'Alessandris QG, De Simone C, et al. Ulnar nerve entrapment at the elbow. A surgical series and a systematic review of the literature. *J Clin Neurosci*. 2017;46:99–108 [Fig. 2].)

down (Fig. 14.12). Tinel sign at the elbow is often present when the ulnar nerve is stimulated. The Wartenberg sign, as well as the Froment, Jeanne, and finger adduction tests, may aid in the diagnosis of tardy ulnar palsy (see Figs. 14.1, 14.4, 14.5, and 14.6).

TESTING

Electromyography with nerve conduction velocity testing is an extremely sensitive test and the skilled electromyographer can diagnose ulnar nerve entrapment at the elbow with a high degree of accuracy—as well as help sort out other neuropathic causes of pain that may mimic ulnar nerve entrapment at the elbow—including radiculopathy and plexopathy (see later). Plain radiographs are indicated in all patients who present with ulnar nerve entrapment at the elbow to rule out occult bony pathology. If surgery is contemplated, an MRI scan of the affected elbow may help further delineate the pathologic process responsible for the nerve entrapment (e.g., bone spur, tumor, or aponeurotic band thickening) (Fig. 14.13; see also Fig. 14.12). If Pancoast tumor or other tumors of the brachial plexus are suspected, chest radiographs with apical lordotic views may be helpful (Fig. 14.14). Screening laboratory testing consisting of complete blood count, erythrocyte sedimentation rate, antinuclear antibody testing, and automated blood chemistry testing should be performed if the diagnosis of ulnar nerve entrapment at the elbow is in question to help rule out other causes of the patient's pain. The injection technique described subsequently will serve as a diagnostic and a therapeutic maneuver.

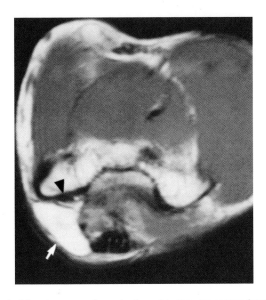

Fig. 14.13 Entrapment of the ulnar nerve *(arrow)* adjacent to the ulnar nerve *(arrowhead)* is well shown in these transverse intermediate-weighted (TR/TE 2000/20) spin echo magnetic resonance (MR) images. The lipoma led to clinical findings of ulnar nerve entrapment in this 36-year-old man. (From Waldman S, Bloch J: *Pain Management*. Philadelphia, PA: Saunders; 2007 [Fig. 66.4].)

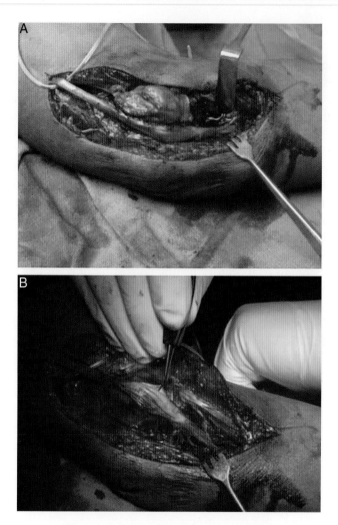

Fig. 14.14 Tardy ulnar palsy findings at surgery. Ulnar nerve thickening at medial epicondyle (A). Epineurolysis of ulnar nerve (B). (From Thiyam R, Lalchandani R. Tardy ulnar nerve palsy after fracture non-union medial epicondyle of humerus—an unusual case. *J Clin Orthop Trauma*. 2015;6(2): 137—139 [Fig. 3].)

DIFFERENTIAL DIAGNOSIS

Ulnar nerve entrapment at the elbow is often misdiagnosed as golfer's elbow, and this fact accounts for the many patients whose "golfer's elbow" fails to respond to conservative measures. Cubital tunnel syndrome can be distinguished from golfer's elbow in that in cubital tunnel syndrome, the maximal tenderness to palpation is over the ulnar nerve 1 inch below the medial epicondyle, whereas with golfer's elbow, the maximal tenderness to palpation is directly over the medial epicondyle. Cubital tunnel syndrome should also be differentiated from cervical radiculopathy involving the C7 or C8 roots and golfer's elbow. It should be remembered that cervical radiculopathy and ulnar nerve entrapment may coexist as the so-called double crush syndrome, which is seen most commonly with median nerve entrapment at the wrist or carpal tunnel syndrome.

TREATMENT

A short course of conservative therapy consisting of simple analgesics, non-steroidal antiinflammatory agents (NSAIDs) or cyclooxygenase-2 (COX-2) inhibitors, and splinting to avoid elbow flexion is indicated in patients who present with ulnar nerve entrapment at the elbow. If the patient does not experience a marked improvement in symptoms within 1 week, careful injection of the ulnar nerve at the elbow using the following technique is a reasonable next step.

Ulnar nerve injection at the elbow is carried out by placing the patient in the supine position with the arm fully adducted at the patient's side and the elbow slightly flexed, with the dorsum of the hand resting on a folded towel. A total of 5 to 7 mL of local anesthetic is drawn up in a 12-mL sterile syringe. A total of 80 mg of depot steroid is added to the local anesthetic with the first block and 40 mg of depot steroid is added with subsequent blocks.

The clinician then identifies the olecranon process and the medial epicondyle of the humerus. The ulnar nerve sulcus between these two bony landmarks is then identified. After preparation of the skin with antiseptic solution, a 0.625-inch, 25-gauge needle is inserted just proximal to the sulcus and is slowly advanced in a slightly cephalad trajectory (Fig. 14.15). As the needle advances approximately 0.5 inch, a strong paresthesia in the distribution of the ulnar nerve will be elicited. The patient should be warned that a paresthesia will occur and to say "there!!!!" as soon as the paresthesia is felt. After paresthesia is elicited and its distribution identified, gentle aspiration is carried out to identify blood. If the aspiration test is negative and no persistent paresthesia into the distribution of the ulnar nerve remains, 5 to 7 mL of solution is slowly injected, with the patient being monitored closely for signs of local anesthetic toxicity. If no paresthesia can be elicited, a similar amount of solution is slowly injected in a fanlike manner just proximal to the notch, with care being taken to avoid intravascular injection. Ultrasound-guided injection may be useful to decrease the incidence of needle-induced complications.

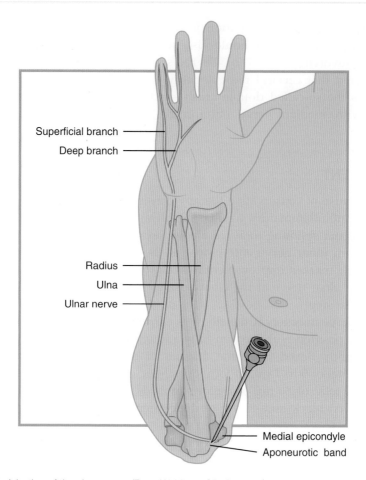

Fig. 14.15 Injection of the ulnar nerve. (From Waldman SD, Bloch J: *Pain Management*. Philadelphia, PA: Saunders; 2007 [Fig. 66.5].)

HIGH-YIELD TAKEAWAYS

- The patient is afebrile, making an acute infectious etiology unlikely.
- The patient's symptomatology is thought to be the result of prolonged pressure on the right ulnar nerve.
- Physical examination and testing should be focused on identification of the various causes of tardy ulnar palsy.
- The patient exhibits the neurologic and physical examination findings highly suggestive of tardy ulnar palsy.

(Continued)

- The patient's symptoms are unilateral, suggestive of a local process rather than a systemic inflammatory process, although the patient has rheumatoid arthritis.
- Plain radiographs will provide high-yield information regarding the bony contents of the joint, but ultrasound imaging and MRI will be more useful in identifying soft tissue pathology that may be responsible for ulnar nerve compromise.
- Electromyography and nerve conduction velocity testing will help delineate the location and degree of nerve compromise if ulnar nerve compromise is suspected.

Suggested Readings

Boone S, Gelberman RH, Calfee RP. The management of cubital tunnel syndrome. *J Hand Surg Am.* 2015;40(9):1897−1904.

Brubacher JW, Leversedge FJ. Ulnar neuropathy in cyclists. *Hand Clin.* 2017;33 (1):199−205.

Shen L, Masih S, Patel DB, et al. MR anatomy and pathology of the ulnar nerve involving the cubital tunnel and Guyon's canal. *Clin Imaging.* 2016;40(2):263−274.

Waldman SD. The little finger adduction test for ulnar nerve entrapment at the elbow. In: *Physical Diagnosis of Pain: An Atlas of Signs and Symptoms.* 4th ed. Philadelphia, PA: Saunders; 2017:134−135.

Waldman SD. The Wartenberg test for ulnar nerve entrapment at the elbow. In: *Physical Diagnosis of Pain: An Atlas of Signs and Symptoms.* 4th ed. Philadelphia, PA: Saunders; 2017:133−134.

Waldman SD. Ulnar nerve entrapment at the elbow. In: *Pain Review.* Philadelphia, PA: Saunders; 2016:270−271.

Mitch Morales

A 38-Year-Old Male With Severe Posterior Elbow Pain

- Learn the common causes of elbow pain.
- Learn the common causes of triceps tendinitis.
- Develop an understanding of the anatomy of the triceps tendon.
- Develop an understanding of the differential diagnosis of triceps tendinitis.
- Learn the clinical presentation of triceps tendinitis.
- Learn how to examine the elbow.
- Learn how to examine the triceps tendon.
- Learn how to use physical examination to identify triceps tendinitis.
- Develop an understanding of the treatment options for triceps tendinitis.

Mitch Morales

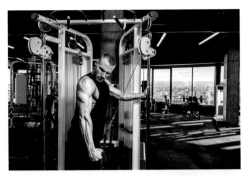

Mitch Morales is a 38-year-old police officer with the chief complaint of, "I can't exercise because my elbow is killing me." Mitch stated that over the last 2 weeks, his right elbow has become increasingly more painful in spite of Advil, topical analgesic balm, and ice packs. He stated that he tried to "burn through it" because he didn't want to "mess with my routine." He noted that the pain was made worse with exercise, specifically with his triceps strengthening exercises. He went on to say, "I can ignore the pain, but my sleep is getting so jacked up. I'm afraid of falling asleep while driving." I asked Mitch if he had ever had anything like this in the past and he said, "Not really, just the usual muscle strains that go along with staying fit." I asked if he was experiencing any numbness and he shook his head. "But you know, Doc, the craziest thing is when I flex and extend my right arm, I get this creaking sensation. It's really weirding me out!" I asked Mitch about any fever, chills, or other constitutional symptoms such as weight loss, night sweats, etc., and he just shook his head no. I then asked Mitch to point with one finger to show me where it hurt the most. He pointed to his right posterior elbow.

On physical examination, Mitch was afebrile. His respirations were 16, his pulse was 66 and regular, and his blood pressure was 112/68. Mitch's head, eyes, ears, nose, throat (HEENT) exam was normal, as was his cardiopulmonary examination. His thyroid was normal. He was well muscled. His abdominal examination revealed no abnormal mass or organomegaly. There was no costovertebral angle (CVA) tenderness. There was no peripheral edema. His low back examination was unremarkable. Visual inspection of the right elbow was unremarkable. There was no rubor and no obvious infection or olecranon bursitis present. Palpation of the posterior elbow revealed some warmth and tenderness over the distal insertion of the triceps tendon. I was able to appreciate crepitus on passive and active resisted flexion and extension over the posterior elbow, consistent with a positive creaking tendon sign (Fig. 15.1). The left elbow examination was normal. A careful neurologic examination of the upper extremities was completely normal. Deep tendon reflexes were normal.

Key Clinical Points—What's Important and What's Not

THE HISTORY

- A history of the onset of right posterior elbow pain associated with use of exercise equipment

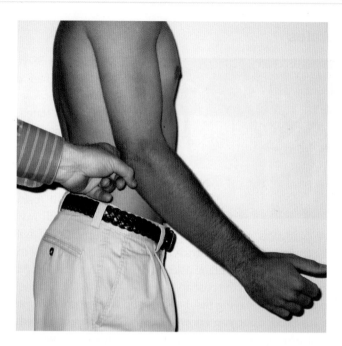

Fig. 15.1 The creaking tendon sign for triceps tendinitis is performed by having the patient extend the affected arm against active resistance while the examiner palpates the distal triceps tendon. (From Waldman SD. *Physical Diagnosis of Pain: An Atlas of Signs and Symptoms*. 3rd ed. St Louis, MO: Elsevier; 2016 [Fig. 83.1].)

- No numbness
- No weakness
- No history of previous significant elbow pain
- No fever of chills

THE PHYSICAL EXAMINATION

- The patient is afebrile
- Crepitus over the triceps tendon on passive and active resisted flexion and extension
- Positive creaking triceps tendon sign
- Warmth over the posterior elbow

OTHER FINDINGS OF NOTE

- Normal HEENT examination
- Normal cardiovascular examination
- Normal pulmonary examination

- Normal abdominal examination
- No peripheral edema
- Normal upper extremity neurologic examination, motor and sensory examination

 ## What Tests Would You Like to Order?

The following tests were ordered:
- Plain radiographs of the right elbow
- Ultrasound of the right elbow
- Magnetic resonance imaging (MRI) of the right elbow

TEST RESULTS

- The plain radiographs of the right elbow revealed tendon and soft tissue calcifications (Fig. 15.2).
- Ultrasound examination of the right elbow revealed partial tearing of the triceps tendon with coexistent tendinitis (Fig. 15.3).
- MRI scan of the right elbow reveals a partial tear of the superficial elements of the right triceps tendon (Fig. 15.4).

 ## Clinical Correlation—Putting It All Together

What is the diagnosis?
- Triceps tendinitis
- Partial tear of the triceps tendon

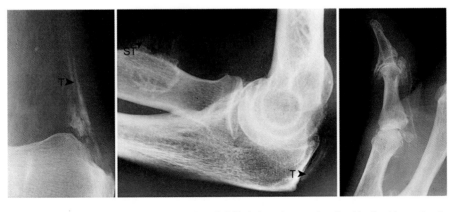

Fig. 15.2 Tendon and soft tissue calcification. Calcified deposits are visualized in the triceps tendon *(T)* and soft tissues *(ST)* around the proximal end of the radius. (From Waldman SD. *Atlas of Uncommon Pain Syndromes*. 3rd ed. Philadelphia, PA: Saunders; 2014 [Fig. 41.1].)

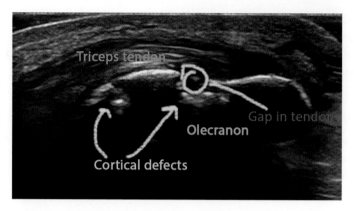

Fig. 15.3   Ultrasound image demonstrating tearing of the triceps tendon. (Courtesy Steven Waldman, MD.)

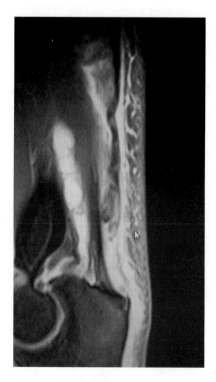

Fig. 15.4   Sagittal magnetic resonance imaging (MRI) of high-grade partial tear of the distal triceps tendon. The superficial tendon is torn, whereas the deep tendon remains intact. *Arrow* points to retracted superficial tendon and surrounding fluid. (From Keener JD, Sethi PM. Distal triceps tendon injuries. *Hand Clin.* 2015;31(4):641–650 [Fig. 7].)

The Science Behind the Diagnosis

ANATOMY

The triceps brachii muscle is a three-headed muscle that serves as the main extensor of the elbow joint and is the antagonist muscle to the biceps brachii and brachialis muscles. Each of the three heads of the triceps muscle has a different origin. The long head of the triceps finds its origin at the infraglenoid fossa of the scapula and receives innervation from the axillary nerve, unlike the rest of the triceps, which is innervated by the radial nerve. The medial head finds its origin at the groove of the radial nerve as well as from the dorsal surface of the humerus, the medial intermuscular septum, and the lateral intermuscular septum. The lateral head finds its origin at the dorsal surface of the humerus at a point lateral and proximal to the groove of the radial nerve as well as the greater tubercle, down to the region of the lateral intermuscular septum. The three heads of the triceps muscle coalesce into the dense distal triceps tendon, which inserts onto the olecranon process and the posterior wall of the capsule of the elbow joint (Fig. 15.5). It is at its point of insertion that the distal triceps musculotendinous unit is susceptible to the development of tendonitis, tears, and rupture (Fig. 15.6).

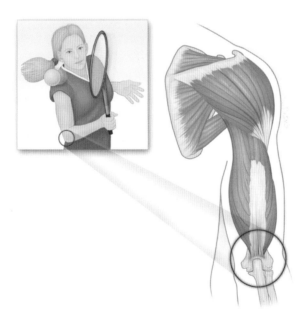

Fig. 15.5 The pain of triceps tendinitis is constant and severe and is localized in the posterior elbow. (From Waldman SD. *Atlas of Uncommon Pain Syndromes*. 3rd ed. Philadelphia, PA: Saunders; 2014 [Fig. 41.3].)

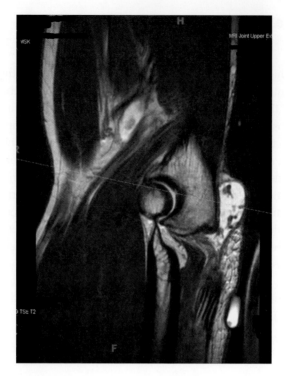

Fig. 15.6 Sagittal T2-weighted magnetic resonance imaging (MRI) of a displaced acute triceps tendon injury; a complete rupture with only a few fibers of the deep central triceps tendon intact. (From Keener JD, Sethi PM. Distal triceps tendon injuries. *Hand Clin*. 2015;31(4):641–650 [Fig. 6].)

CLINICAL SYNDROME

Triceps tendinitis is being seen with increasing frequency in clinical practice as exercising and the use of exercise equipment have increased in popularity. The triceps tendon is susceptible to the development of tendinitis at its distal portion and its insertion on the ulna. The triceps tendon is subject to repetitive motion that may result in microtrauma, which heals poorly because of the tendon's avascular nature. Exercise is often implicated as the inciting factor of acute triceps tendinitis. Tendinitis of the triceps tendon frequently coexists with bursitis of the associated bursae of the tendon and elbow joint, creating additional pain and functional disability. Calcium deposition around the tendon may occur if the inflammation continues, making subsequent treatment more difficult (see Fig. 15.2). Continued trauma to the inflamed tendon ultimately may result in tendon rupture (Fig. 15.7).

SIGNS AND SYMPTOMS

The onset of triceps tendinitis is usually acute, occurring after overuse or misuse of the elbow joint. Inciting factors include playing tennis and

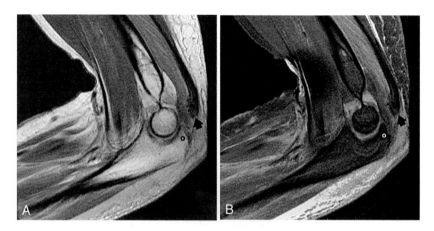

Fig. 15.7 Triceps tendon rupture imaged in flexion. This patient was unable to extend the elbow because of discomfort. The images were obtained on a high-field scanner with the patient prone and the arm flexed overhead. Proton density (A) and fat-suppressed T2-weighted (B) coronal images reveal a fluid-filled tear of the distal triceps tendon *(arrows)* from the olecranon *(O)*. (From Waldman SD. *Atlas of Uncommon Pain Syndromes*. 3rd ed. Philadelphia, PA: Saunders; 2014 [Fig. 41.2].)

aggressive use of exercise machines. Improper stretching of triceps muscle and triceps tendon before exercise also has been implicated in the development of triceps tendinitis and acute tendon rupture. Injuries ranging from partial to complete tears of the tendon can occur when the distal tendon sustains direct trauma while it is fully flexed under load or when the elbow is forcibly flexed while the arm is fully extended. The pain of triceps tendinitis is constant and severe and is localized in the posterior elbow. Significant sleep disturbance is often reported. Patients with triceps tendinitis exhibit pain with resisted extension of the elbow. A creaking or grating sensation may be palpated when passively extending the elbow. As mentioned, a chronically inflamed triceps tendon may rupture suddenly with stress or during vigorous injection procedures inadvertently injected into the substance of the tendon. With triceps tendon rupture, the patient is unable to fully and forcefully extend the affected arm.

TESTING

Plain radiographs, ultrasound imaging, and MRI are indicated for all patients who present with posterior elbow pain (see Figs. 15.2–15.4). Based on the patient's clinical presentation, additional tests, including complete blood count, erythrocyte sedimentation rate, and antinuclear antibody testing, may be indicated. MRI of the elbow is indicated if joint instability is suspected and to confirm the diagnosis. Radionuclide bone scanning is useful to identify stress fractures of the elbow not seen on plain radiographs.

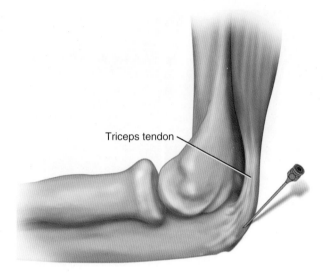

Fig. 15.8   Injection technique for triceps tendinitis. (From Waldman SD. *Atlas of Pain Management Injection Techniques*. 4th ed. St Louis, MO: Elsevier; 2017 [Fig. 57.6].)

DIFFERENTIAL DIAGNOSIS

Triceps tendinitis generally is easily identified on clinical grounds, but coexistent bursitis may confuse the diagnosis. Stress fractures of the olecranon also may mimic triceps tendinitis and may be identified on plain radiographs or radionuclide bone scanning.

TREATMENT

Initial treatment of the pain and functional disability associated with triceps tendinitis should include a combination of nonsteroidal antiinflammatory drugs (NSAIDs) or cyclooxygenase-2 (COX-2) inhibitors and physical therapy. The local application of heat and cold also may be beneficial. Patients should be encouraged to avoid repetitive activities responsible for the evolution of the tendinitis. For patients who do not respond to these treatment modalities, injection with local anesthetic and steroid may be a reasonable next step (Fig. 15.8).

HIGH-YIELD TAKEAWAYS

- The patient is afebrile, making an acute infectious etiology unlikely.
- The patient's symptomatology is thought to be the result of overuse injury to the right triceps tendon.

(Continued)

- Physical examination and testing should be focused on identification of the various causes of triceps tendinitis.
- The patient exhibits physical examination findings that are highly suggestive of triceps tendinitis.
- The patient's symptoms are unilateral, suggestive of a local process rather than a systemic inflammatory process, although the patient has rheumatoid arthritis.
- Plain radiographs will provide high-yield information regarding the bony contents of the joint, but ultrasound imaging and MRI will be more useful in identifying soft tissue pathology that may be responsible for triceps tendon compromise.

Suggested Readings

Badia A, Stennett C. Sports-related injuries of the elbow. *J Hand Ther*. 2006;19:206–227.

Isbell WM. Tendon ruptures. In: Brukner P, Khan K, eds. *Clinical Sports Medicine*. 3rd ed. Sydney: McGraw-Hill; 2006.

Jafarnia K, Gabel GT, Morrey BF. Triceps tendinitis. *Oper Tech Sports Med*. 2001;9:217–221.

Keener JD, Chafik D, Kim HM, et al. Insertional anatomy of the triceps brachii tendon. *J Shoulder Elbow Surg*. 2010;19:399–405.

Rineer CA, Ruch DS. Elbow tendinopathy and tendon ruptures: epicondylitis, biceps and triceps ruptures. *J Hand Surg Am*. 2009;34:566–576.

Waldman SD. Ultrasound-guided injection technique for triceps tendinitis. In: *Comprehensive Atlas of Ultrasound Guided Pain Management Injection Techniques*. Philadelphia, PA: Lippincott; 2014. 388–385.

Functional anatomy of the elbow. In: Waldman SD, ed. *Pain Review*. Philadelphia, PA: Saunders; 2009:76–77.

INDEX

Page numbers followed by '*f*' indicate figures, '*t*' indicate tables.